WJ168

Reconstructive Surgery of the Lower Urinary Tract in Children

Provided as a service to urology by

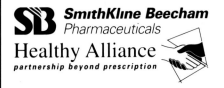

SmithKline Beecham
Pharmaceuticals
Healthy Alliance
partnership beyond prescription

Reconstructive Surgery of the Lower Urinary Tract in Children

Edited by

Joachim W. Thüroff MD

Professor and Chairman, Department of Urology, Klinikum Barmen, University of Witten/Herdecke Medical School, Heusnerstrasse 40, 42283 Wuppertal, Germany

and

Markus Hohenfellner MD

Associate Professor of Urology, Department of Urology, Klinikum Barmen, University of Witten/Herdecke Medical School, Heusnerstrasse 40, 42283 Wuppertal, Germany

I S I S
MEDICAL
MEDIA

Oxford

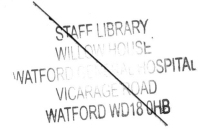

British Library Cataloguing in Publication Data.
A catalogue record for this title is available from
the British Library

ISBN 1 899066 16 0

Thüroff J. W. (Joachim)
Reconstructive Surgery of the Lower Urinary Tract in Children/
Joachim W. Thüroff and Markus Hohenfellner

Always refer to the manufacturer's Prescribing
Information before prescribing drugs cited in this book.

Set by
Creative Associates, Oxford, England

Printed by
Dah Hua Printing Press Co. Limited, Hong Kong

Distributed by
Times Mirror International Publishers
Customer Service Centre, Unit 1, 3 Sheldon Way
Larkfield, Aylesford, Kent, ME20 6SF
UK

Contents

CONTENTS

List of Contributors

Terry D. Allen MD
Professor of Urology, Department of Urology, University of Texas Southwestern Medical Center, Children's Medical Center, 1935 Motor Street, Dallas, Texas 75235, USA

Kaname Ameda MD
Department of Urology, Hokkaido University School of Medicine, Kita 15-jo, Nishi 7-chome, Kita-ku, Sapporo 060, Japan

Sami Arap MD
Full Professor and Chairman, Division of Urology, Hospital das Clínicas, Sao Paulo University School of Medicine, Av. Dr. Enéas de Carvalho Aguiar, 225-a/710F,05403-000, Sao Paulo - SP, Brazil

Yoshifumi Asano MD
Department of Urology, Hokkaido University School of Medicine, Kita 15-jo, Nishi 7-chome, Kita-ku, Sapporo 060, Japan

Anthony Atala MD
Division of Urology, Children's Hospital, 300 Longwood Avenue, Boston, Massachusetts 02115, USA

Yoshiaki Banya MD
Assistant Professor of Urology, Department of Urology, Iwate Medical University School of Medicine, 19-1 Uchimaru, Morioka 020, Japan

Joseph Barone MD
Division of Urology, Emory University, 1901 Century Boulevard NE, Suite 14, Atlanta, Georgia 30345, USA

Adair J. Batista MD
Department of Urology, Universidade Federal de Uberlandia, Urologia Clinica, Av. Getulio Vargas 295, C.P. 605, Uberlandia MG, 38401.001, Brazil

Stuart B. Bauer MD
Division of Urology, Children's Hospital, 300 Longwood Avenue, Boston, Massachusetts 02115, USA

Bruce H. Broecker MD FACS FAAP
Division of Urology, Emory University , 1901 Century Boulevard NE, Suite 14,
Atlanta, Georgia 30345, USA

Rainer Bürger MD
Associate Professor, Department of Urology, University of Mainz Medical School,
Langenbeckstrasse 1, 55131 Mainz, Germany

Michael C. Carr MD
Division of Urology, Children's Hospital, 300 Longwood Avenue, Boston,
Massachusetts 02115, USA

Arnold H. Colodny MD
Division of Urology, Children's Hospital, 300 Longwood Avenue, Boston,
Massachusetts 02115, USA

Michael Cher MD
Department of Urology, UCSF Medical Center, 533 Parnassus, San Francisco,
California 94143, USA

A. Dickson MD
Department of Paediatric Urology, Royal Manchester Children's Hospital, Hospital
Road, Pendlebury, Manchester, M27 4HA, UK

Zdeněk Dítě MD
Assistant Professor of Urology, Division of Urology, Postgraduate Medical School
Prague, Ke Karlova 6, 120 00 Praha 2, Czech Republic

Jan Dvořáček MD DrSc
Professor of Urology, Clinic of Urology, First Faculty of Medicine, Charles
University Prague, Ke Karlovu 6, 120 00 Praha 2, Czech Republic

David H. Ewalt MD
Assistant Professor of Urology, Department of Urology, University of Texas
Southwestern Medical Center, Children's Medical Center, 1935 Motor Street, Dallas,
Texas 75235, USA

Wouter Feitz MD
Department of Urology, University Hospital Nijmegen, Postbox 9101, 6500 HB
Nijmegen, The Netherlands

Margit Fisch MD
Department of Urology, University of Mainz Medical School, Langenbeckstrasse 1,
55131 Mainz, Germany

Tomoaki Fujioka MD
*Department of Urology, Iwate Medical University School of Medicine, 19-1
Uchimaru, Morioka 020, Japan*

Amilcar M. Giron MD
*Associate Professor of Pediatric Urology, Division of Urology, Hospital das Clínicas,
Sao Paulo University School of Medicine, Av. Dr. Enéas de Carvalho Aguiar, 225-
a/710F,05403-000, Sao Paulo - SP, Brazil*

Rafael Gosalbez Jr MD
Division of Urology, University of Miami, Miami, Florida, USA

David C.S. Gough FRCS FRACS DCH
*Consultant Paediatric Urologist, Department of Paediatric Urology, Royal Manchester
Children's Hospital, Hospital Road, Pendlebury, Manchester, M27 4HA, UK*

Eiji Higashihara MD
*Professor and Chairman, Department of Urology, Kyorin University School of
Medicine, 6-20-2 Shinkawa, Mitaka-shi, Tokyo, 181, Japan*

Rudolf Hohenfellner MD
*Professor and Chairman, Department of Urology ,University of Mainz,
Langenbeckstrasse 1, 55131, Mainz, Germany*

Edson Ide MD
*Department of Urology, Universidade Federal de Uberlandia, Urologia Clinica, Av.
Getulio Vargas 295, C.P. 605, Uberlandia MG, 38401.001, Brazil*

Koichi Ishikura MD
*Department of Urology, Iwate Medical University School of Medicine, 19-1
Uchimaru, Morioka 020, Japan*

Ladislav Jarolím MD PhD
*Associate Professor of Urology, Clinic of Urology, First Faculty of Medicine, Charles
University Prague , Ke Karlovu 6, 120 00 Praha 2, Czech Republic*

Tsuneo Kajikawa MD
*Department of Urology, Iwate Medical University School of Medicine, 19-1
Uchimaru, Morioka 020, Japan*

Hidehiro Kakizaki MD
*Department of Urology, Hokkaido University School of Medicine, Kita 15-jo Nishi
7-chome, Kita-ku, Sapporo 060, Japan*

Dae Kyung Kim MD
*Senior Resident, Department of Urology, Seoul National University Children's
Hospital, 28 Yunkun-Dong, Chongno-Gu, Seoul, 110-744, Korea*

Kwang M. Kim MD
*Associate Professor, Department of Urology, Seoul National University Children's
Hospital, 28 Yunkun-Dong, Chongno-Gu, Seoul, 110-744, Korea*

Lowell R. King MD FACS
*Division of Urologic Surgery, Duke University Medical Center, P.O. Box 3707,
Durham, North Carolina 27710, USA*

George T. Klauber MD
*Department of Pediatric Urology, New England Medical Center, 750 Washington
Street, Box 92, Boston, Massachusetts 02111, USA*

Shinya Kobayashi MD
*Department of Urology, Hokkaido University School of Medicine, Kita 15-jo, Nishi
7-chome, Kita-ku, Sapporo 060, Japan*

Radim Kočvara MD PhD
*Clinic of Urology, General Teaching Hospital Prague , Ke Karlovu 6, 120 00 Praha
2, Czech Republic*

Tomohiko Koyanagi MD
*Professor and Chairman, Department of Urology, Hokkaido University School of
Medicine, Kita 15-jo, Nishi 7-chome, Kita-ku, Sapporo 060, Japan*

Milos Kralj MD
*Consultant and Head of Urology Department, University Medical Centre, Zaloska 7,
61000 Ljubljana, Slovenia*

Takashi Kubo MD
*Department of Urology, Iwate Medical University School of Medicine, 19-1
Uchimaru, Morioka 020, Japan*

Takashi Kurosawa MD
*Department of Urology, Iwate Medical University School of Medicine, 19-1
Uchimaru, Morioka 020, Japan*

Ahnkie Lee MD
*Chief, Department of Urology, Seoul City Boramae Hospital, #395 Shindaebang-
Dong, Dongjak-Gu, Seoul 156-100, Korea*

LIST OF CONTRIBUTORS

Edward J. McGuire MD
Professor of Surgery (Urology), Department of Urology, University of Texas-Houston, 6431 Fannin, 6.018, Houston, Texas, 77030, USA

James Mandell MD
Division of Urology, Children's Hospital, 300 Longwood Avenue, Boston, Massachusetts 02115, USA

Charlotte A. Massad MD
Division of Urology, Emory University , 1901 Century Boulevard NE, Suite 14, Atlanta, Georgia 30345, USA

Kinya Matsumura MD
Department of Urology, Hokkaido University School of Medicine, Kita 15-jo, Nishi 7-chome, Kita-ku, Sapporo 060 , Japan

Junichi Matsuzaka MD
Department of Urology, Iwate Medical University School of Medicine, 19-1 Uchimaru, Morioka 020, Japan

Jan Nijhuis MD
Department of Gynaecology, University Hospital Nijmegen, Postbox 9101, 6500 HB Nijmegen, The Netherlands

Katsuya Nonomura MD
Associate Professor, Department of Urology, Hokkaido University School of Medicine, Kita 15-jo, Nishi 7-chome, Kita-ku, Sapporo 060, Japan

Akimi Ogawa MD
Professor and Chairman, Department of Urology, Shinshu University School of Medicine, 3-1-1- Asahi, Matsumoto 390, Japan

Thomas S. Parrott MD FACS FAAP
Division of Urology, Emory University , 1901 Century Boulevard NE, Suite 14, Atlanta, Georgia 30345, USA

Luis M. Pérez MD
Division of Urology, Emory University , 1901 Century Boulevard NE, Suite 14, Atlanta, Georgia 30345, USA

Craig A. Peters MD
Division of Urology, Children's Hospital, 300 Longwood Avenue, Boston, Massachusetts 02115, USA

Neilton G. Prado MD
Professor and Chairman, Department of Urology, Universidade Federal de Uberlandia, Urologia Clinica, Av. Getulio Vargas 295, C.P. 605, Uberlandia MG, 38401.001, Brazil

Alan B. Retik MD
Professor of Surgery (Urology), Harvard Medical School; Chief, Division of Urology, Children's Hospital, 300 Longwood Avenue, Boston, Massachusetts 02115, USA

Richard N. Schlussel MD
Division of Urology, Children's Hospital, 300 Longwood Avenue, Boston, Massachusetts 02115, USA

Koji Seino MD
Department of Urology, Iwate Medical University School of Medicine, 19-1 Uchimaru, Morioka 020, Japan

Takashi Shibata MD
Department of Urology, Hokkaido University School of Medicine, Kita 15-jo, Nishi 7-chome, Kita-ku, Sapporo 060, Japan

Yuichiro Shinno MD
Department of Urology, Hokkaido University School of Medicine, Kita 15-jo, Nishi 7-chome, Kita-ku, Sapporo 060, Japan

Edwin Smith MD
Fellow, Division of Urology, Emory University, 1901 Century Boulevard NE, Suite 14, Atlanta, Georgia 30345, USA

Franz Spies MD
Department of Urology, University of Mainz Medical School, Langenbeckstrasse 1, 55131 Mainz, Germany

Raimund Stein MD
Resident, Department of Urology, The University of Mainz Medical School , Langenbeckstrasse 1, 55131 Mainz, Germany

Michael Stöckle MD
Associate Professor, Department of Urology, University of Mainz Medical School, Langenbeckstrasse 1, 55131 Mainz, Germany

Fujio Takakura MD
Department of Urology, Hokkaido University School of Medicine, Kita 15-jo, Nishi 7-chome, Kita-ku, Sapporo 060, Japan

Bojan Tršinar MD
Urological Clinic, University Medical Centre Ljubljana, Zaloska 7, 61000 Ljubljana, Slovenia

Thomas Tsang MD
Department of Paediatric Urology, Royal Manchester Children's Hospital, Hospital Road, Pendlebury, Manchester, M27 4HA, UK

Joseph D. de Vries MD
Associate Professor, Department of Urology, University Hospital Nijmegen, P.O. Box 9101, 6500 HB Nijmegen, The Netherlands

Robert Wammack MD
University of Mainz, Department of Urology, Langenbeckstrasse 1, 55131, Mainz, Germany

Kenji Watanabe MD
Associate Professor, Department of Urology, Shinshu University School of Medicine, 3-1-1- Asahi, Matsumoto 390, Japan

Michel de Wildt MD
Department of Urology, University Hospital Nijmegen, P.O. Box 9101, 6500 HB Nijmegen, The Netherlands

John R. Woodard MD FACS FAAP
Division of Urology, Emory University, 1901 Century Boulevard N.E. Suite 14, Atlanta, Georgia 30345, USA

Christopher R. J. Woodhouse MB FRCS
Senior Lecturer, The Institute of Urology; Consultant Urologist, St. George's Hospital; Honorary Consultant Urologist, The Hospital for Sick Children, Great Ormond Street, London, UK

Daniel Yachia MD
Head, Department of Urology, Hillel Yaffe Medical Center, Hadera 38100, Israel ; Israel Lecturer, Sackler Medical School, University of Tel Aviv, Tel Aviv, Israel.

Tetsufumi Yamashita MD
Department of Urology, Hokkaido University School of Medicine, Kita 15-jo, Nishi 7-chome, Kita-ku, Sapporo 060, Japan

Preface

This volume of the SIU series constitutes the Proceedings of the 23rd congress of the Société Internationale d' Urologie (SIU) held in Sydney, Australia from 18 to 22 September 1994, on the major topic of the congress: 'Reconstructive Surgery of the Lower Urinary Tract in Children'. The volume has been assembled from the papers presented in the main session on this topic and from selected additional papers presented in other oral and poster sessions of the congress.

The arrangement of papers in this volume reflects the structure of the SIU congress: the keynote reviews from Sydney are presented as state-of-the-art reports and each is matched with original contributions from the scientific programme on the same subject as that report.

The topics that are discussed deal with hypospadias repair, penile and urinary reconstruction in exstrophy and epispadias, enterocystoplasty and urinary diversion in exstrophy and neuropathic bladder and other means of treatment of neuropathic bladder. The result of such an assembly is a kaleidoscope of current opinions on diagnosis, pathophysiology, aetiology, research and therapy throughout the world of urology.

The ingenuity of urologists in developing new techniques of plastic reconstruction seems to be unlimited, as demonstrated by the fascinating and exciting examples of alternative techniques for hypospadias repair. However, in the hands of the individual surgeon, standardization and perfection of a technique may play an even more important part in increasing success rates and lowering complication rates than the specific technique selected. Thus, many of the techniques presented may be considered to be variations of a limited number of basic principles of plastic surgery applied to urethral and penile reconstruction. Whenever the surgical technique adheres to the correct basic principles and pays attention to detail, surgeons may achieve very similar results with differing techniques. It is the beauty of SIU congresses (which, it is hoped, is reflected in this volume) that experts worldwide share their expertise, not only for the interest and pleasure of presenting the variety and spectrum of this specialty but also for teaching and learning, one from another. If this book can contribute to the latter aspect, its aim will have been achieved.

Joachim W. Thüroff   Markus Hohenfellner

REPORT

Hypospadias repair

1

T. Koyanagi   K. Nonomura   H. Kakizaki
T. Yamashita

Introduction

Repair of the deformity of hypospadias is one of the most challenging issues in paediatric reconstructive surgery. First, the structures concerned are small. This is not only age related but also inherent in this disorder, in which there may be constitutional small size or endocrinological hypogonadism.[1-3] A multiplicity of anomalies may need reconstruction, ranging from hypospadiac urethra, chordee, or a globular glans with dorsal skin hood, to a bifid scrotum in very severe cases. The impact of genital surgery and its sequelae on the subsequent psychological development of boys, particularly when multistage or complex surgery is necessary, must also be considered.[4] This report reviews the problems encountered in hypospadias repair and presents the authors' experience of one-stage repair.

Classification

Traditionally, this has been based on the anatomical location of the meatus, which is classified as glanular, subcoronal, penile, penoscrotal, scrotal or perineal.[5] The meatus is often relocated after the release of chordee or correction of ventriflexion.[6] For this reason, Duckett prefers a classification relating to the new location of the meatus after the curvature has been released, in which anterior, middle and posterior hypospadias are designated.[7] The authors advocate the classification system of distal and proximal hypospadias, in which the location of the meatus is assessed with reference to (i.e. whether distal or proximal to) the penoscrotal junction[8,9] (Table 1.1).

Aetiological considerations

Normally, the urethral groove is formed into a tube by the epithelial fusion of the urethral folds in the ventral midline, proximally to distally, during weeks 7–14 of gestation. The tubular urethra becomes invested by the mesenchyme, the future corpus spongiosum. Labioscrotal folds, which

Duckett	Traditional	Koyanagi
Anterior	Glanular (meatus situated on the inferior surface of the glans)	
	Coronal (meatus situated in the balanopenile furrow)	
	Anterior penile (meatus situated in the distal third of the shaft)	Distal
Middle	Middle penile (meatus situated in the middle third of the shaft)	
Posterior	Posterior penile (meatus situated in the posterior third of the shaft)	
	Penoscrotal (meatus situated at the base of the shaft in front of the scrotum)	
	Scrotal (meatus situated on the scrotum or between the genital swellings)	Proximal
	Perineal (meatus situated behind the scrotum or behind the genital swellings)	

Table 1.1. Classification of hypospadias with modification according to Duckett[7]

are lateral to the urethral plate and anterior to the genital tubercle (which is a cylindrical phallus at this stage), begin their caudal migration, with subsequent midline fusion and formation of the scrotum. This process of fusion of the urethral folds and subsequent coverage with ventrally migrated penile skin and subcutaneous tissue extends to the glans penis. At this period of development the glans contains the urethral plate, a lamina of epithelium lacking a lumen.

During the final embryogenesis of the anterior urethra between weeks 12 and 16 of gestation, the glanular urethra is formed by the fusion of glanular folds proximally to distally, while the epithelial tag and core at the tip of the glans and about the urethra canalize. Along with the formation of the glanular urethra, its floor is covered by ventrally migrated preputial folds and then with glanular mesenchyme, which before this time had existed as a distinct structure from the corpus spongiosum or corpus cavernosum, thus bringing about frenular and glanular fusion in the midline. During this process the prepuce forms by overgrowing the glans owing to proliferation of the penile skin and subcutaneous tissue. By the time that the abutting wall disintegrates, the glanular urethra is infiltrated with its own mesenchyme as the spongy urethra and opens as the external meatus. When complete, the glans, which was previously ventrally tilted and globular, attains its normal cone shape with a vertically slit meatus at the most distal end of the glans.[10,11]

This formation of the anterior urethra, which is part of the normal masculinization process of the external genitalia in boys,[12] is somehow jeopardized in cases of hypospadiac penis. Absence of the corpus spongiosum beyond the urethral orifice has been observed in some cases of hypospadias.[13-15] Thus, the failure of fusion of the urethral folds, and subsequent inadequate condensation of mesenchymal tissue, may be attributable to the arrested development of the epithelium of the urethra, and subsequently of the corpus spongiosum,[16] in severe proximal hypospadias[14,15] (Fig. 1.1). In less severe — and most cases of distal — hypospadias, the presence of the corpus spongiosum dorsolateral and distal to the urethral orifice has been confirmed.[17-19] This corpus spongiosum is deficient ventrally by being splayed out laterally, but it is not fibrotic[20] (Fig. 1.2). These findings suggest an abnormal embryogenesis, in the form of incomplete fusion of the urethral folds in the presence of mesenchymal infiltration of the future corpus spongiosum.

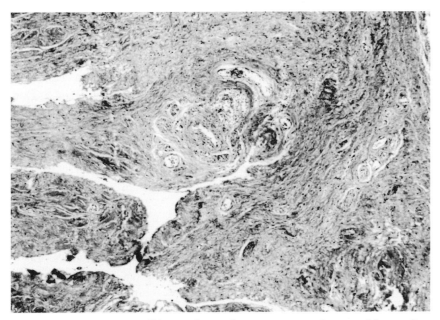

Figure 1.1. Tissue specimen of hypospadiac urethra in a patient with proximal hypospadias. Only a tiny remnant of spongy tissue is visible among abundant dysplastic connective tissue.

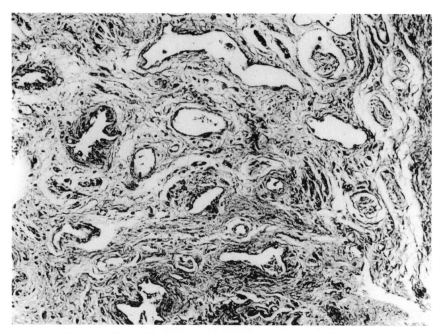

Figure 1.2 Histopathology of hypospadiac urethra in a patient with distal hypospadias. The urethra is not atretic or dysplastic, but contains normal spongy tissues rich in capillaries with abundant smooth musculature.

The exact mechanism of the defective embryogenesis remains speculative. Pituitary and gonadal function in prepubertal boys with hypospadias is found to be more deficient in the proximal than in the distal type,[1,2] suggesting a failure of androgenic stimulation to complete the formation of the urethra and migration of the scrotal and penile foreskin. Maternal progestin during a critical embryofoetal stage is also implicated as a possible cause of hypospadias.[2,21] Nevertheless, the precise cause of hypospadias is still unknown. It is probably polygenic, in view of its higher familial incidence.[7]

Associated anomalies

In the authors' experience of 61 children with hypospadias, 36 (59%) were found to have concurrent genitourinary anomalies.[3] Of these 36 children, 17 cases (47%) had abnormal scrotal contents (undescended testes in ten, monorchidism in one, dysgenetic testes in one, hydrocoele in five); in 13 cases (36%) there were lower urinary tract anomalies (utriculus masculinus in 11 and meatal stricture in two), 11 (31%) had anomalies involving the scrotum and penis (propenile scrotum in nine, microphallus in one, penile torsion in one) and four (11%) had renal and ureteral anomalies (fused kidney, renal malrotation, duplex, and ureteral reflux, respectively). A similar incidence of undescended testes and/or utricle has been reported by others,[22,23] and there is an increasing tendency to the latter with increasing severity of hypospadias.[24] In view of the normal masculinization process under the endocrinological influence of the pituitary and testis, the high incidence of concurrent genital anomalies is not surprising as a deficiency of androgenic stimulation is also implicated in these anomalies.[12,25] The lower incidence of urinary tract anomalies may be due to the fact that the external genitalia are formed much later than the supravesical portion of the urinary tract.[7] The lower rate (1–4.6%) reported by others makes further urinary tract evaluation unnecessary.[22,26]

The incidence of anomalies other than those of the genitourinary system was 14 cases (39%) (inguinal hernia, eight cases, ventricular and atrial septal defect, three cases and one case respectively, and auricular defect, two cases). An unusual concurrence of Wilms' tumour, nephrosis and hypospadias with male intersex suggested the Drash syndrome.[27] The recorded birth weight of 59 of the children with hypospadias ranged from 1200 to 3900 g (mean 2846 g). There were 16 (27%) premature children with low birth weight (<2500 g) for date.[3]

Features of the hypospadias anomaly

Meatus and glans
The urethral meatus may be only slightly ventrally placed just below a blind dimple at the glans (an infranavicular hypospadias), or the urethra may be set back in the perineum. In infranavicular hypospadias a bridge of tissue is present between the blind dimple and the meatus, representing a remnant of the abutment between the canalized epithelial core distally and glanular folds proximally during the final stage of glanular urethral formation.[28] Often there is an orifice of a periurethral duct distal to the meatus which corresponds to Guérin's sinus or Morgani's lacunae[29] (Fig. 1.3). Although the meatus is located in any part of the transitional zone from perineum to glans, the glans becomes flattened and globular as the meatus recedes proximally. This change in glanular shape, from conical to globular, is a reflection of defective ventral migration of the glanular mesenchyme, which becomes fused in the midline over the glanular urethra.[11,30]

Dorsal skin hood and bifid scrotum
In hypospadias there is a failure not only of the urethral folds to fuse but also of the labioscrotal swellings and preputial folds to do so by migrating ventrally over the bulbar and spongy urethra.[10] Subsequently, the scrotal

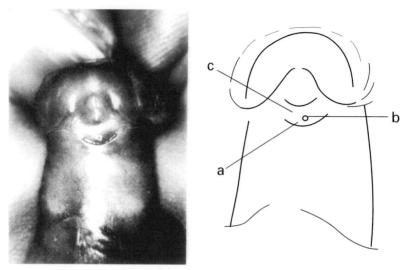

Figure 1.3. Ventral aspect of glans and penile shaft in distal hypospadias. The meatus (a), which in this case slightly resembles a megameatus, is located in the anterior penile shaft. Just distal to it is the orifice (b) of a periurethral duct. A bridge of tissue (c) between the meatus and the cleaved glans represents the junction between the anterior urethra and glanular urethra.

and penile foreskin adheres to both sides of the hypospadiac urethra. This results in a varying degree of propenile scrotum (scrotal transposition) or bifid scrotum and skin hood surmounting the dorsalis of the penis (Fig. 1.4).

Curvature

Abnormal ventral curvature of the penis has been termed 'chordee', as this implies a strand of connective tissue stretched like a cord between the meatus and glans. Mettauer,[31] in 1842, described this cord as a rudiment of the urethral corpus spongiosum,[14–16] to which the penile shaft adheres together with the scrotal and phallic skin, hindering their free sliding, with a resultant ventral curvature or bowing of the shaft. This hypothesis is supported by the fact that the mammalian spongy urethra requires androgenic stimulation for its development;[32] this is significantly impaired in severe hypospadias,[2] as discussed in the section on aetiology and may explain the presence of chordee.

In distal and less severe hypospadias, the urethra is not rudimentary or fibrously atretic but its spongy tissue is splayed out distally,[17–19] lacking Buck's fascia and loose subcutaneous tissue. Skin adheres not only to the edges of the hypospadiac urethra but also most prominently to the ventral part of the urethral wall proximal to the hypospadiac meatus.[18] Thus, if the skin is incised along a line encircling the meatus proximally

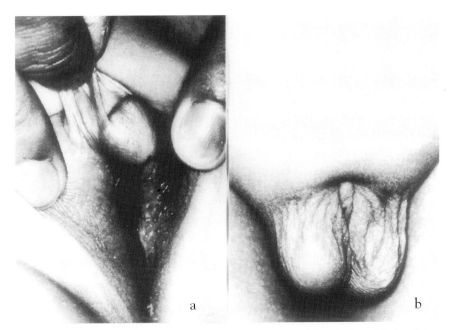

Figure 1.4. Dorsal appearance of penis and scrotum in proximal hypospadias: (a) dorsal skin hood and severe chordee (ventriflexion of penis); (b) bivalved scrotum apparent as a propenile scrotum.

and extending dorsolaterally and circumferentially parallel to the sulcus coronalis, its subsequent mobilization in the plane between Buck's fascia and the dartos fascia (dartos mobilization) usually restores the curvature and free sliding of the penile shaft. The lack of contribution of the urethral plate to chordee is easily confirmed by creation of an artificial erection.[8,20] In any case, this adhesion of skin and its investing Buck's and dartos fasciae to the hypospadiac urethra is a significant factor in the formation of the penile curvature in hypospadias.

Other causes of curvature include different rates of growth of the normal dorsal phallic tissue and the abnormal ventral urethral plate,[33] and an asymmetric degree of distensibility of the tunica albuginea between the dorsal and ventral aspect of the corpora.[34,35]

A physiological ventral curvature of the penis, which has been documented at different stages of foetal development but usually disappears by birth, may be found in premature infants.[36] Incomplete investment of the periurethral fascia has been suggested as a cause of ventral curvature in chordee without hypospadias.[37] Prematurity or low birth weight is a common finding among children with hypospadias.[3] Overall, deficient periurethral fascial cover may have a role in these children in a setting of prematurity.[38]

7

Repair of hypospadias

Ever since surgeons started to undertake repair of hypospadias early in this century, the field has been studded with numerous varieties of different methods. In 1968, Culp and McRoberts reviewed more than 150 reputedly original methods of urethral reconstruction,[39] to which it is reported that another 50 have subsequently been added.[7] Several elements of the abnormalities call for meticulous repair: thus the surgical repair may include orthoplasty (or chordectomy), urethroplasty, glanulomeatoplasty, skin coverage and scrotoplasty.[7] Current trends are directed to younger patients and fewer operations with minimum hospitalization; this is becoming a reality owing to progress in 'hypospadiology'.[40] Nevertheless, in this section, multistage repair is first reviewed and then the one-stage method is described, with particular emphasis on the authors' technique of single-stage repair.

Multistage repair

Initially, penile curvature is corrected. This chordectomy (orthoplasty) is accomplished by dividing the urethral plate at the point of greatest curvature distal to the meatus, straightening the penis, and allowing the meatus to retract to a more proximal position. Boisson (1861) was the first to suggest a transverse incision at the point of greatest curvature.[41] The dorsal foreskin is then transposed to cover the ventrum of the penile corpora, either by formation of a buttonhole[42] or using Byars' technique.[43]

At least 6 months after the first stage of repair, when skin healing is complete, a second stage of repair is undertaken to reconstruct the urethra using the ventrally transposed penile foreskin. The principal methods of urethroplasty are the buried strip described by Browne[5,44] or the urethral tube devised by Thiersch in 1869[45] and Duplay in 1874.[41] The buried strip never gave very satisfactory results; van der Meulen[46] demonstrated that a rotated skin cover from the dorsum with an eccentric suture line would bring about more successful healing.

The concept of tubularizing the urethra, as advocated by Thiersch (1869)[45] and Duplay (1874),[41] rather than the use of a buried strip to form the new urethra, was initiated by Byars,[43] and popularized by Smith,[47] Belt and Fuqua,[48] and Hendren.[49] To bring the urethral orifice to the tip of the glans, the glans splitting technique of Beck[50] and Barcat[51] was used,[43,47] or the glans was chanelled by removing a core of substance to pass the neourethra.[49,52]

Scrotoplasty for scrotal transposition is usually reserved for the final (third) stage,[6] using various techniques.[44,53,54]

One-stage repair

In 1900, Russell[55] described a procedure using a urethral tube constructed from a flap that was developed on the ventral surface of the penis. This flap extended around the entire circumference of the corona to include a cuff of the prepuce. Unfortunately, this pioneering work of urethroplasty immediately following orthoplasty in a combined one-stage repair was considered to be doomed to failure[56] (which was far from being the case)[57–59] and has met with little acceptance. Others — Humby in 1941[60] and Davis in 1951[61] — continued to perfect the technique, and yet their success was not accepted or at least could not be emulated by their colleagues.[7] In the early 1960s a renewal of interest in one-stage repair was initiated by a number of surgeons;[62–64] this culminated in the further development of other techniques in the late 1960s[65] and 1970s.[66–68]

In association with these new techniques, revised concepts of the genesis of chordee or ventral curvature[17–19] and the development of the artificial erection technique,[69] which has almost eliminated inadequate chordee release, paved the way for further technical refinements[19,20,34,70–74] and the firm establishment of the one-stage repair of hypospadias in the current practice of paediatric reconstructive surgery. Specific techniques for surgical repair of varying types of hypospadias have been delineated by Duckett.[7] He has stressed that a great deal depends on experience, but even more on familiarity with all the options available. Indeed, with this familiarity as a prerequisite he has proposed 'hypospadiology' as an appropriate term for this discipline.[40]

One-stage urethroplasty with parameatal foreskin-flap (OUPF): a simple method universally applicable to all types of hypospadias

Numerous operative techniques have been reported for the repair of hypospadias. Those who tackle this difficult and challenging problem have long been advised to be well acquainted with a variety of such techniques. The one-stage repair that has evolved over the past two decades is now in vogue and has withstood the test of time;[7] in the majority of cases of distal hypospadias, remarkably high success rates can be expected with a variety of types of single-stage repair.[68,70,75] None the less, in the repair of proximal hypospadias, in which the deformity is much more severe, these techniques have a limited role, and only a few have been established as suitable for correction of all the concurrent abnormalities (e.g. hypospadiac urethra with severe chordee, ventrally tilted globular glans with dorsal skin hood, and propenile bifid scrotum) in one stage with a reasonable rate of success;[54,76] many still advise staged repair in this difficult setting.[7] Admittedly, the repair of hypospadias is one of the most complex and demanding procedures of reconstructive urological surgery and the advice that hypospadiologists should be well armed with all these operative techniques as their options is well taken. Nevertheless, a simple single-stage method that is universally applicable to all types of hypospadias, from very mild (glanular and coronal) and moderate (penile and distal to penoscrotal) to more severe ones (scrotal and perineal), would immensely benefit both these children and the hypospadiologists alike. In the authors' opinion, the technique of one-stage urethroplasty with parameatal foreskin flap (OUPF)[77] conforms to these criteria.

Operative technique

Basically, the technique follows steps 1–7 summarized in Fig. 1.5.

Step 1: outlining the skin incision and dartos mobilization. Independent of the type of hypospadias, an encircling skin incision is made proximal to the meatus and extending dorsolaterally, including sufficient parameatal foreskin (Fig 1.6a, b; Fig. 1.7, step 1; Fig 1.8a, b; Fig. 1.9, step 1).

Step 2: Artificial erection, harvesting parameatal foreskin flap(s), and chordectomy as needed. After dartos mobilization and artificial erection, if chordee is absent, as in most cases of distal hypospadias,[18] an adequate length of flap is harvested from either side of the parameatal foreskin (Fig. 1.6c–f; Fig. 1.7, step 2). If chordee is present, as in most cases of proximal hypospadias, flaps are harvested from both sides of the parameatal foreskin and joined by transecting the urethral plate. The urethra with bilateral parameatal foreskin flaps is detached from the ventralis of the corpora, as in classic chordectomy, until the shaft straightens (Fig. 1.8c–g; Fig. 1.9, step 2).

Step 3: Glans cleavage and creation of glanular wings. When chordee is absent at the outset, or has been released by dartos mobilization alone, an incision is made, parallel to both sides of the urethral groove, and the glans is cleaved, thus preserving the urethral plate (Fig. 1.6f, g; Fig. 1.7, step 3). When the urethra is severed, the glans is cleaved by a vertical midline incision. After the glans has been split thus, the incision is deepened to the level of the corpora and glanular wings are created by judicious lateralization of the glanular substance, literally 'kippering' the glans (i.e. splitting it and splaying it out laterally, to flatten it; Fig. 1.8h–j; Fig. 1.9, step 3).[78] Because of the separate origins of the glans, urethra and corporal body,[10,11] this dissection can usually be accomplished anatomically without undue bleeding.

Step 4: OUPF. When the urethral plate is preserved, the parameatal foreskin flap is simply laid on top of it to form the neourethra (OUPF-II) (Fig. 1.6h; Fig. 1.7, step 4).[8] When the urethral plate is transected and severed, the neourethra is formed by tubularizing the bilateral parameatal

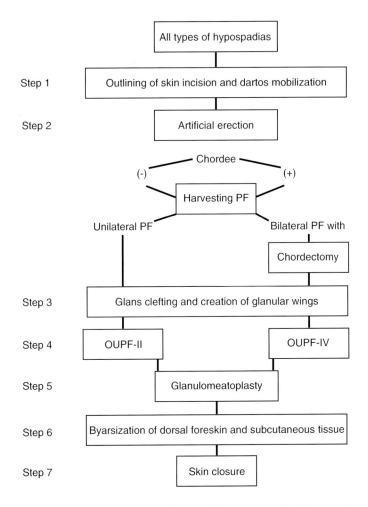

Figure 1.5. Flowchart of operative technique. PF, parameatal foreskin flap; OUPF, one-stage urethroplasty with parameatal foreskin flap; (–), chordee released, (+), chordee remaining.

foreskin flaps and is anchored to the tip of the 'kippered' glans (OUPF-IV).[9] Owing to the urethral mobilization at chordectomy (step 2) there should not be any tension on anchoring the neourethra to the glans (Fig. 1.8k–m; Fig. 1.9, step 4).

Step 5: Glanulomeatoplasty. The glans wings are approximated over the neourethra as well as the paraglanular foreskin to cover the glanular and frenular portion of the distal urethra, while the rest of the somewhat protruding urethral edge is everted and sutured to the glanular edge in a semicuffed fashion. When completed, a vertically slip meatus opens at the most distal end of the glans which has been restored to a normal

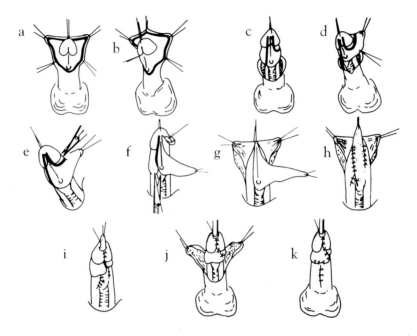

Figure 1.6. Schematic illustrations of the technique of onlay urethroplasty with parameatal foreskin flap (OUPF-II). A detailed description is given in reference 8.

conical shape from being somewhat ventrally tilted and globular (Fig 1.6i; Fig 1.7, step 5; Fig. 1.8n–p; Fig 1.9, step 5).

Step 6: 'Byarsization'. Byars' technique[43] is applied to the dorsal foreskin and its subcutaneous tissue (Fig 1.6j; Fig 1.7, step 6; Fig. 1.8q–s; Fig. 1.9, step 6).

Step 7: Skin closure. This is shown in Fig. 1.6k, Fig. 1.7, step 7, Fig. 1.8t–w and Fig. 1.9, step 7. Steps 6 and 7 are essentially the same as reported previously,[8,9] although it should again be stressed that, in proximal hypospadias (in which propenile bifid scrotum is often a concurrent abnormality), at step 1 it is mandatory to mobilize the scrotum extensively, and at step 6 its subcutaneous tissue is also 'byarsized' sufficiently to reposition it ventral and posterior to the penile shaft, thus rectifying this abnormality also.[9] For the specific details of each step the reader is referred to the originals[8,9] and the American Urological Association (AUA) videolibrary series.[79]

Postoperative care

All patients are managed with urethral drainage using a fine (6 Fr) indwelling silicone catheter (Cliny® Create Medic, Japan) which is left *in situ* for 1 week (in OUPF-II) to 2 weeks (in OUPF-IV). The other management procedures including wound dressing and after removal of the catheter, are as reported previously.[8,9]

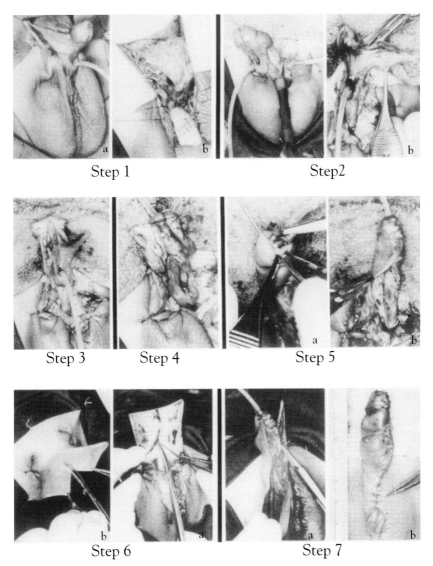

Figure 1.7. Photographic illustrations of the technique of onlay urethroplasty with parameatal foreskin flap (OUPF-II). A detailed description is given in reference 8.

Results

A total of 120 patients have been subjected to this technique over the past 10 years; their ages ranged from 2 to 12 years (mean of 3.7 years). OUPF-II was advocated in 50 cases and OUPF-IV in 70. One-third of those patients undergoing OUPF-IV were those in whom dartos mobilization alone was insufficient to restore the chordee in apparently distal hypospadias, and who were converted intraoperatively to undergo

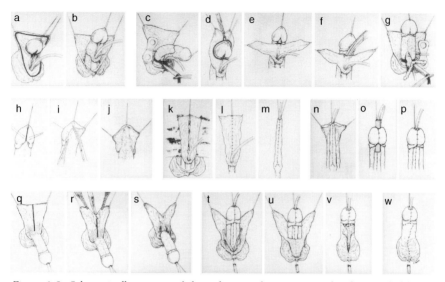

Figure 1.8. Schematic illustrations of the technique of one-stage urethroplasty with bilateral parameatal foreskin flaps (OUPF-IV). Details are given in reference 9.

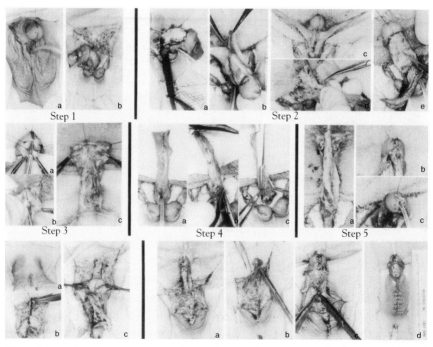

Figure 1.9. Photographic illustrations of the technique of one-stage urethroplasty with bilateral parameatal foreskin flaps (OUPF-IV). Details are given in reference 9.

OUPF-IV. In 70 cases there was a primary cure without complications. A small fistula occurred in eight cases, but all healed, with expectant treatment, within 2 months. Including these cases, primary success was obtained in 82% (41/50) with OUPF-II and 53% (37/70) with OUPF-IV. Complications requiring secondary repair occurred in 42 cases: these comprised meatal stricture requiring recession or glanular dehiscence with meatal recession in 15 (three with OUPF-II and 12 with OUPF-IV), urethrocutaneous fistula in 21 cases (six with OUPF-II and 15 with OUPF-IV) and urethral stricture in six cases (all with OUPF-IV). Secondary procedures were done in 32 cases (extension urethroplasty in 15 and fistula closure in 17 cases), attaining satisfactory results in 29 cases. Thus the overall success rate is 91% [96% (48/50) with OUPF-II and 87% (61/70) with OUPF-IV]. Both functional and cosmetic outcome were satisfactory with either technique (Fig. 1.10). Eleven patients are awaiting additional repair (eight secondary, two tertiary, and one quaternary).

Comments
As discussed in the section describing the features of hypospadias, chordee is either absent or is relieved by dartos mobilization alone;

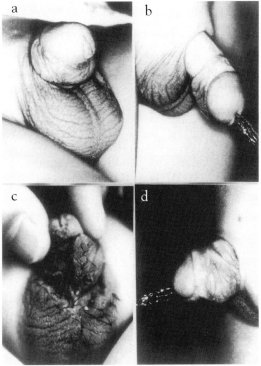

Figure 1.10. Outcome of OUPF-II (a,b) and OUPF-IV (c,d).

however, it is difficult to predict the severity of chordee preoperatively. In glanular or coronal hypospadias it is absent in most cases, enabling repair to be undertaken by the MAGPI[70] (meatoplasty and glanuloplasty) and/or flip-flap techniques.[65] In other types of hypospadias, distal to penoscrotal, dartos mobilization alone is often adequate to alleviate chordee,[18] thus clearing the way for various types of one-stage repair with preservation of the urethral plate.[66,74] Artificial erection under anaesthesia before the skin incision may be helpful in selecting the operation of choice, but seems cumbersome. Furthermore, in hypospadias that is apparently distal to penoscrotal, dartos mobilization alone fails to relieve chordee in one-third of cases.[77] Nevertheless, urethral mobilization[20,80,81] or dorsal tunica albuginea plication of the corpora, as judiciously utilized by Baskin et al.,[35] may prove beneficial; if this is of no avail, then it is necessary to transect the urethra before carrying out what is currently the most reliable one-stage repair procedure using a transverse preputial island flap urethroplasty for proximal hypospadias.[54,82] Faced with the possibility of encountering these unexpected situations, the hypospadiologist is well advised to be armed with various technical options.[7] Nevertheless, a simple method applicable to all types of hypospadias should be available.

The OUPF technique described in this chapter is unique in this regard. The planned skin incision that is necessary in most repair procedures is not required, except at the initial skin incision (step 1), which is essentially the same no matter what the type or severity of hypospadias. The technique differs only at step 4. After dartos mobilization, basically there are only two methods for formation of the neourethra (OUPF-II and OUPF-IV), the choice of which is made on the basis of artificial erection. Allowing this intraoperative choice of either OUPF-II or OUPF-IV, depending on the degree of chordee remaining, considerably simplifies the procedure and enables all types of hypospadias to be tackled with confidence. The viability of a parameatal foreskin flap, even in a setting of OUPF-IV, is well established.[8] It also has considerably better microcirculatory parameters than the meatal-based ventral midline flap, which is why OUPF-II is preferred by the authors, in which the MAGPI or flip-flap technique is probably indicated. The neourethra is in natural continuity with the old urethra, allowing less risk of complication at their junction. Urethras constructed in this way continue to grow, as seen in the oldest of the children (now over 13 years of age) treated by the authors. Compared with the glans-piercing technique, this glanulomeatoplasty appears to be embryologically as well as anatomically more sound,[10,11] and it is instrumental in obtaining a cosmetically and functionally satisfactory result. Moreover, on skin closure the propenile scrotum can be repositioned ventral and posterior to the penile shaft, thus enabling substantial correction of concurrent anomalies to be made, even in the severest forms of hypospadias, all in one stage. The OUPF technique should be added to the hypospadiologist's armamentarium as a simple and yet reliable one-stage method of correction of all types of hypospadias, with a reasonable rate of success.

Conclusions

Hypospadia is a severe anomaly, the repair of which was previously a formidable task, even with multistage operations. In the last two decades, however, great progress has been made both in the basic understanding of this deformity and in its surgical repair, which has culminated in the discipline aptly termed 'hypospadiology'.[7] In 1941, Higgins wrote in a prophetic foreword: 'If, however, one could succeed in remodeling the urethra in one operation, the gain would be manifest.'[60] This now seems to be a reality. Much of the current success is attributable to delicate tissue handling, the basic principles of plastic surgery, excellent microscopic instruments and materials, improved perioperative and postoperative care and numerous other factors.

In the authors' experience, the long-term outcome of single-stage repair has been satisfactory, both functionally and cosmetically. Incomplete chordee release has been eliminated by assessment with artificial erection. The reconstructed urethra grows with the patient. On puberty, most of the testicular deficiency[2] appears to become normalized and testicular function shows a sudden increase. Psychological anxiety, which was the probable outcome of multistage operations, is now less of a problem with the single-stage operation, although a recent analysis has reported that, in some cases of severe proximal hypospadias, psychosomatic adjustment has been poor.[83] Nevertheless, nowadays parents of the majority of children with hypospadias can be counselled with optimism and confidence;[7] the day has come when all types of hypospadias are amenable to complete repair in a single-stage operation with a reasonable rate of success.

References

1. Allen T D, Griffin J E. Endocrine studies in patients with advanced hypospadias. J Urol 1984; 131: 310–314
2. Nonomura K, Fujieda K, Sakakibara N et al. Pituitary and gonadal function in prepubertal boys with hypospadias. J Urol 1984; 132: 595–598
3. Sakakibara N, Nonomura K, Matsuno T, Koyanagi T. Some clinical and endocrinological study of hypospadias. Jpn J Urol 1985; 76: 716–722

4. Berg R, Svensson J, Astrom G. Social and sexual adjustment of men operated for hypospadias during childhood: a controlled study. J Urol 1981; 125: 313–317

5. Browne D. An operation for hypospadias. Lancet 1936; 1: 141–143

6. Barcat J. Current concepts of treatment. In: Horton C E (ed) Plastic and reconstructive surgery of the genital area. Boston: Little, Brown, 1973: 249–263

7. Duckett J W. Hypospadias. In: Walsh P C , Retik A B, Stamey T A, Vaughan E D, Jr (eds) Campbell's Urology, 6th ed. Philadelphia: Saunders, 1992: 1893–1910

8. Koyanagi T, Nonomura K, Asano Y et al. Onlay urethroplasty with parameatal foreskin flap for distal hypospadias. Eur Urol 1991; 19: 221–224

9. Koyanagi T, Nonomura K, Kakizaki H et al. Experience with one-stage repair of severe proximal hypospadias: operative technique and results. Eur Urol 1993; 24: 106–110

10. Altemus A R, Hutchins G M. Development of the human anterior urethra. J Urol 1991; 146: 1085–1093

11. Stephens F D, Fortune D W. Pathogenesis of megalourethra. J Urol 1993; 149: 1512–1516

12. Walsh P C, Migeon C J. The phenotypic expression of selective disorders of male sexual differentiation. J Urol 1988; 119: 627–629

13. Devine C J Jr. Embryology of the male external genitalia. Clin Plast Surg 1980; 7: 141–148

14. Koyanagi T. Repair of severe proximal hypospadias associated with bifid scrotum. Int Urol Nephrol 1984; 16: 115–121

15. Marshall M Jr, Johnson S H, Price S E Jr et al. Cecil urethroplasty with concurrent scrotoplasty for repair of hypospadias. J Urol 1979; 121: 335–338

16. Williams D I. The development and abnormalities of the penile urethra. Acta Anat 1952; 15: 176–187

17. Smith D R. Repair of hypospadias in the preschool child: a report of 150 cases. J Urol 1967; 97: 723–730

18. Marshall M Jr, Beh W P, Johnson S H III et al. Etiologic consideration in penoscrotal hypospadias repair. J Urol 1978; 120: 229 231

19. Koyanagi T. Modification of the King–Hoffman urethroplasty for one-stage repair of distal shaft penile hypospadias. Int Urol Nephrol 1984; 16: 219–225

20. Koyanagi T, Matsuno T, Nonomura K, Sakakibara N. Complete repair of severe penoscrotal hypospadias in 1 stage: experience with urethral mobilization, wing flap-flipping urethroplasty and 'glanulomeatoplasty'. J Urol 1983; 130: 1150–1154

21. Aarskog D. Maternal progestins as a possible cause of hypospadias. New Engl J Med 1989; 300: 75–78

22. Khuri F J, Hardy B E, Churchill B M. Urologic anomalies associated with hypospadias. Urol Clin North Am 1981; 8: 565–571

23. Bauer S B, Retik A B, Colodny A H. Genetic aspects of hypospadias. Urol Clin North Am 1981; 8: 559–564

24. Shima H, Ikoma F, Terakawa T et al. Developmental anomalies associated with hypospadias. J Urol 1979; 122: 619–621

25. Rajfer J, Walsh P C. Hormonal regulation of testicular descent: experimental and clinical observations. J Urol 1977; 118: 985–990

26. McAndle F, Lebowitz R. Uncomplicated hypospadias and anomalies of upper urinary tract. Need for screening? Urology 1975; 5: 712–716

27. Koyanagi T, Hirama M, Taniguchi K et al. Wilms tumor and nephrotic syndrome in male pseudohermaphroditism. Urology 1984; 24: 595–600

28. Glenister J W. The origin and fate of the urethral plate in man. J Anat 1954; 288: 413–418
29. Sommer J T, Stephens F D. Dorsal urethral diverticulum of the fossa navicularis: symptoms, diagnosis and treatment. J Urol 1980; 124: 94–98
30. Turner-Warwick R. Observation upon techniques for reconstruction of the urethral meatus, the hypospadiac glans deformity and the penile urethra. Urol Clin North Am 1979; 6: 643–655
31. Mettauer J P. Practical observations on those malformations of the male urethra and penis, termed hypospadias and epispadias, with an anomalous case. Am J Med Sci 1842; 4: 43–57
32. Nonomura K, Sakakibara N, Demura T et al. Androgen binding activity in the spongy tissue of mammalian penis. J Urol 1990; 144: 152–155
33. Bellinger M F. Embryology of the male external genitalia. Urol Clin North Am 1981; 8: 375–382
34. Nesbit R M. Congenital curvature of the phallus: report of three cases with description of corrective operation. J Urol 1965; 93: 230–232
35. Baskin L S, Duckett J W, Ueoka K et al. Changing concepts of hypospadias curvature lead to more onlay island flap procedures. J Urol 1994; 151: 191–197
36. Kaplan G W, Lamm D L. Embryogenesis of chordee. J Urol 1975; 114: 767–773
37. Devine C J Jr, Horton C E. Chordee without hypospadias. J Urol 1973; 110: 264–267
38. Sakakibara N, Nonomura K, Togashi M, Koyanagi T. Experience with 11 cases of chordee without hypospadias. Jpn J Urol 1988; 79: 1555–1558
39. Culp O S, McRoberts J W. Hypospadias. In: Alken C E, Dix V W, Goodwin W et al. (eds) Encyclopedia of urology. New York: Springer-Verlag, 1968: 11307–11344
40. Duckett J W. Foreword: Symposium on Hypospadias. Urol Clin North Am 1981; 8: 371–373
41. Horton C E, Devine C J, Baran N. Pictorial history of hypospadias repair techniques. In: Horton CE (ed) Plastic and recontructive surgery of the genital area. Boston: Little, Brown, 1973: 237–248
42. Nesbit R M. Plastic procedure for correction of hypospadias. J Urol 1941; 45: 699–702
43. Byars L T. A technique for consistently satisfactory repair of hypospadias. Surg Gynecol Obstet 1955; 100: 184–190
44. Browne D. A comparison of the Duplay and Denis Browne techniques for hypospadias operation. Surgery 1953; 34: 787–793
45. Thiersch C. Ueber die Entstehungsweise und operative Behandlung der Epispadie. Arch Heilkunde 1869; 10: 20
46. Van der Meulen J C. Hypospadias monograph. Leiden, The Netherlands: 1964; Stenfert Kroese, NV
47. Smith E D. Durham–Smith repair of hypospadias. Urol Clin North Am 1981; 8: 451–455
48. Fuqua F. Renaissance of urethroplasty: the Belt technique of hypospadias repair. J Urol 1971; 106: 782–785
49. Hendren W H. The Belt–Fuqua technique for repair of hypospadias. Urol Clin North Am 1981; 8: 431–450
50. Beck C. Hypospadias and its treatment. Surg Gynecol Obstet 1917; 24: 511–532
51. Barcat J. Current concepts of treatment. In: Horton C E (ed) Plastic and recontructive surgery of the genital area. Boston: Little, Brown, 1973: 249–263
52. Duckett J W. Hypospadias. Clin Plast Surg 1980; 7: 149–160

53. Glenn J F, Anderson E E. Surgical correction of incomplete penoscrotal transposition. J Urol 1973; 110: 603–605

54. Ehrlich R M, Scardino P T. Surgical correction of scrotal transposition and perineal hypospadias. J Pediatr Surg 1982; 17: 175–177

55. Russell R H. Operation for severe hypospadias. Br Med J 1900; 2: 1432–1435 (cited in ref. 56)

56. Creevy C D. The correction of hypospadias: a review. Urol Surv 1958; 8: 2–68

57. Koyanagi T, Imanaka K, Nonomura K et al. Further experience with one-stage repair of severe hypospadias and scrotal transposition. Modifications in the technique and its result in eight cases. Int Urol Nephrol 1988; 20: 167–177

58. Nonomura K, Koyanagi T, Sakakibara N. A new technique for skin closure in hypospadias: ipsilateral penoscrotal approximation for closure. Urol Int 1987; 42: 309–312

59. Koyanagi T, Nonomura K, Gotoh T et al. One-stage repair of perineal hypospadias and scrotal transposition. Eur Urol 1984; 10: 364–367

60. Humby G. A one-stage operation for hypospadias. Br J Surg 1941; 29: 84–92

61. Davis D M. Surgical treatment of hypospadias, especially scrotal and perineal. J Urol 1951; 65: 595–602

62. Ricketson G A. A method of repair for hypospadias. Am J Surg 1958; 95: 279–283

63. Broadbent T R, Woolf R M, Toksu E. Hypospadias: one-stage repair. Plast Reconstr Surg 1961; 27: 154–157

64. Des Prez J D, Persky L, Kiehn C L. A one-stage repair of hypospadias by island flap technique. Plast Reconstr Surg 1961; 28: 405–410

65. Allen T D, Spence H M. The surgical treatment of coronal hypospadias and related problems. J Urol 1968; 100: 504–508

66. King L R. Hypospadias — a one-stage repair without skin graft based on a new principle: chordee is sometimes produced by skin alone. J Urol 1970; 103: 660–662

67. Hodgson N B. A one-stage hypospadias repair. J Urol 1970; 104: 281–284

68. Devine C J Jr, Horton C E. Hypospadias repair. J Urol 1977; 118: 188–193

69. Gittes R F, McLaughlin A P III. Injection technique to induce penile erection. Urology 1974; 4: 473–475

70. Duckett J W. MAGPI (meatoplasty and glanuloplasty): a procedure for subcoronal hypospadias. Urol Clin North Am 1981; 8: 513–520

71. Gonzales E T Jr, Veeraraghavan K A, Delaune J. The management of distal hypospadias with meatal-based, vascularized flaps. J Urol 1983; 129: 119–120

72. Hodgson N B. Use of vascularized flaps in hypospadias repair. Urol Clin Am 1981; 8: 471–482

73. Duckett J W. The island flap technique for hypospadias repair. Urol Clin North Am 1981; 8: 503–511

74. Elder J S, Duckett J W, Snyder H M. Onlay island flap in the repair of mid and distal penile hypospadias without chordee. J Urol 1987; 138: 376–379

75. Wacksman J, Sheldon C, King L R. Distal hypospadias repair. In: Webster G, Kirby R, King L, Goldwasser B (eds) Reconstructive urology, 1st ed. Oxford: Blackwell Scientific Publications, 1993: 749–762

76. Woodard J R, Parrot T S. Management of severe perineal hypospadias with bifid scrotum. J Urol 1991; 145: 245A (abstr)

77. Koyanagi T, Nonomura K, Asano Y. One-stage urethroplasty with parameatal foreskin flap (OUFP): simple method universally applicable to all types of hypospadias repair. J Urol 1992; 147: 317A (abstr)

78. Turner-Warwick R. Hypospadiac and epispadiac retrievoplasty. In: Webster G, Kirby R, King L, Goldwasser B (eds). Reconstructive urology. 1st ed. Oxford: Blackwell Scientific Publications, 1993; 781–793

79. Nonomura K, Koyanagi T, Kakizaki H et al. One-stage urethroplasty with parameatal foreskin flap for all types of hypospadias. (87th Annual Meeting of American Urological Association, Washington D.C.). J Urol 1992; 147: 188A (videotape V-1)

80. Mollard P, Mouriquand P, Felfela T. Application of the onlay island flap urethroplasty to penile hypospadias with severe chordee. Br J Urol 1992; 68: 317–319

81. Monfort G, Bretheau D, di Benedetto V, Bankole R. Posterior hypospadias repair: a new technical approach. Mobilization of the urethral plate and Duplay urethroplasty. Eur Urol 1992; 22: 137–141

82. Duckett J W. Transverse preputial island flap technique for repair of severe hypospadias. Urol Clin North Am 1980; 7: 423–431

83. Eberle J, Überreiter S, Radmayr C et al. Posterior hypospadias: long-term follow-up after reconstructive surgery in the male direction. J Urol 1993; 150: 1474–1477

2 One-stage repair of severe hypospadias using a bladder mucosal graft and distal glanuloplasty

L. R. King

Introduction

Bladder mucosal grafts were first used to form the requisite length of neourethra in the late 1940s to early 1950s,[1,2] but were largely abandoned because of a high incidence of stricture and meatal prolapse and stenosis.[2,3] When urologists began to visit China more than a decade ago, they found the procedure in general use there and it came into use again in the Western world.[4] However, meatal stenosis, often recurrent, remained a serious problem. Ransley suggested that a small free segment of foreskin be used to form the distalmost portion of the urethra, but such small grafts are difficult to stabilize.[5]

For over 20 years the author has retained the thin mucosa-like skin between the meatus and the corona in older boys, correcting residual chordee from behind after degloving the penis.[6] Undoubtedly, such skin grows as the child grows. It is therefore an easy step to preserve this skin as it is detached from the underlying corpora cavernosa to correct chordee. It should be left attached at the corona, and it is tubularized to form the distal portion of the neourethra. The bladder graft is used to bridge the urethral defect between native meatus and corona, and all of the unrolled dorsal hood is then available to resurface the ventral aspect of the penile shaft. Whereas strictures, occurring commonly at the proximal anastomotic site with the native meatus and where the bladder mucosa is exposed on the glans, previously limited the use of the procedure,[2,3,7] the author has found that draining both anastomoses prevents most strictures. When the distalmost portion of the neourethra is formed from the skin of the ventral penile shaft and glans, no bladder mucosa is exposed, and meatal stricture is thereby avoided.

Patients and methods

Four boys with very proximal hypospadiac openings and severe chordee were judged suitable for this procedure. The foreskin did not appear adequate for both formation of the neourethra and coverage of the ventral penile shaft after the chordee had been completely corrected. Each operation was performed as a planned one-stage repair. In one patient the scrotum was bifid distal to the meatus. A strip of the non-hairbearing skin separating the two halves of the scrotum was used to form the most proximal portion of the neourethra in this instance. The proximal end of the tubularized bladder graft was then anastomosed to the end of the urethra formed from this skin strip, as to the native meatus.

Technique

Chordee must first be completely corrected, making an incision to deglove the penis. In these cases the transverse ventral portion of this incision is as far proximal on the penile shaft as possible, centred just distal to the meatus (Fig. 2.1). The distal skin on the ventrum of the penis is elevated from the underlying corpora to allow it to slide forward to be used as the distalmost portion of the neourethra.[8]

The penis is degloved, and an artificial erection is performed to assess residual chordee. When the shaft of the penis is angulated, the dorsal neurovascular pedicle is mobilized to permit excision of one or two symmetrical transverse wedges of Buck's fascia. The openings in the

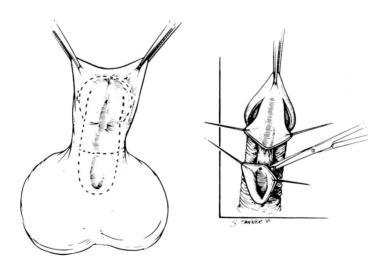

Figure 2.1. The penis is degloved, leaving the skin of the ventral penile shaft attached to the corona. After ventral buried tissue causing chordee has been excised, residual chordee is corrected by removing dorsal transverse wedges of Buck's fascia after mobilization of the dorsal vessels and nerves. Glanular tilt may also require dorsal correction (see text). The skin on the ventral aspect of the penile shaft is preserved to form the distal portion of the neourethra (inset). (Reproduced from ref. 13 with permission.)

corpora cavernosa are closed with close 3/0 chromic catgut sutures, and the artificial erection is repeated.[4] Another wedge can be removed, if needed, without shortening the penis to a measurable degree. When only glanular tilt remains, the space between the glans and the dome of the corpora cavernosa is entered dorsally. Dissection is continued until 1 cm of the raw surface of the glans is exposed. Dexon® sutures (4/0) are then placed absolutely symmetrically between the raw exposed surface of the glans and Buck's fascia. The author usually uses a midline stitch and one on either side. When these have been tied, the artificial erection should be repeated to ensure that the glanular tilt is adequately corrected and that the glans is not angulated laterally.

If the penis is straight, the length of bladder mucosa needed is obtained next. The distance between the detached native urethra and the distal urethral plate is measured. Bladder grafts do not contract, so a graft of this length and 1.6–2 cm wide, depending on the size of the child, is harvested. The graft is outlined with brilliant green or marked with stay sutures to indicate length and width. The graft is then excised with tenotomy scissors, tapering it at either end to facilitate bladder closure. A suprapubic tube is usually inserted, to be used for urinary diversion together with the drip tube. The mucosal surface is turned inward and rolled into a tube with two layers of running locking 5/0 chromic sutures over a stent of appropriate size, usually 12 or 14 Fr, which will be positioned just inside the bladder neck to become a drip tube. The proximal end of the drip tube is subsequently threaded into the urethra, and the graft is orientated so that the suture line is dorsal, against the corpora. The proximal end of the graft is anastomosed to the native meatus, using interrupted 5/0 chromic sutures in two layers, making the anastomosis as watertight as possible.[8,10]

The distal urethral plate is tubularized over the drip tube to form the distalmost neourethra, and the glanuloplasty is completed. The strip of glans forming the glanular urethra is tapered slightly at the neomeatus to make a 'nozzle'. The incisions in the glans should be deep, so the lateral glans flaps are not undermined and their blood supply impaired. The glans flaps are then drawn under the new meatus with interrupted sutures (Fig. 2.2). If there seems to be tension on the glans flap, the glanular urethra can be covered with transposed foreskin. The urethroplasty is completed by anastomosing the distal end of the bladder graft to the distalmost urethra formed from the ventral penile skin.

The entire dorsal hood has been preserved to resurface the ventral aspect of the penile shaft. The dorsal hood is unrolled, and handled with traction sutures. Since van der Meulen showed that the foreskin is drained by a single vein, the author has usually preferred his technique of

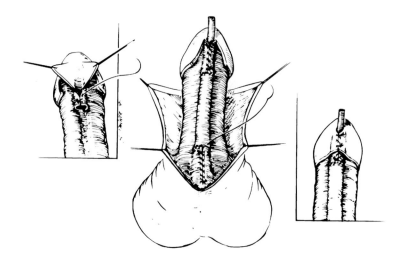

Figure 2.2. The tubularized bladder graft is orientated with the suture line against the corpora. Two-layer, watertight anastomoses are then made to the native meatus and to the preserved penile skin and glanuloplasty. (Reproduced from ref. 13 with permission.)

foreskin transposition (Fig. 2.3).[9,10] The dorsal hood is divided asymmetrically to the base of the foreskin at the dorsal midpoint. Thus the entire foreskin has good venous drainage and the transposed major flap covers the neourethra with overlapping suture lines only at the corona. Alternatively, Byars' flaps may be employed.[11] The drip tube is carefully positioned so that the end is just inside the bladder and is sewn to the glans with two 2/0 silk sutures. Small Penrose or TLS drains are placed alongside the anastomotic sites and exit from the base of the penis. A Tegaderm® dressing is applied to the penis, and a light pressure dressing to the scrotum to prevent excessive oedema. Belladonna and opium suppositories are used prophylactically every 4–6 h to prevent bladder spasms, and antibiotics are continued for 3 days, after which sulfisoxazole is given. The drip tube is kept in place for 7–10 days, and if it is working well the drains are removed on day 3. The suprapubic tube is clamped to permit voiding, the day after the drip tube is removed.

Results

Mean follow-up is 2 years and 4 months. Three of the four boys healed per primum, had satisfactory cosmetic results and have not required reoperation. No meatal stenosis has occurred. The third of the four patients in this series had a sizeable fistula, 8 mm in diameter, at the

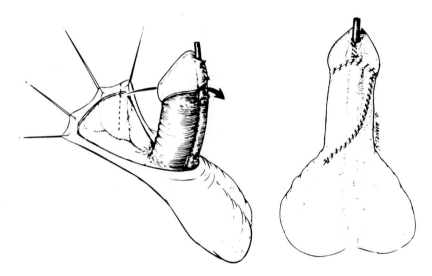

Figure 2.3. Van der Meulen's technique of foreskin transposition. The dorsal hood is unrolled and the large central vein identified. An incision is made from the distal edge of the foreskin on one side to the base of the foreskin at the midline, creating flaps of unequal size. The major flap is transposed across the midline. The incision at the base of the transposed foreskin may be extended to provide a pleasing cosmetic appearance, but the subcutaneous pedicle must be preserved. (Reproduced from ref. 13 with permission.)

corona. After healing was complete this was successfully circumscribed, closed in two layers and covered with a skin flap derived from the ventral aspect of the penile shaft proximally. A small scrotal flap was used to close the donor site. No patient has experienced persistent or recurrent chordee.

Discussion

The author has had extensive experience using the 'urethral plate', the mucosa-like skin between the native meatus and the glans, to form the neourethra when chordee can be corrected by degloving the penis, with or without correction of residual chordee by wedge resection of the dorsal corpora cavernosa.[6] It is simple, conceptually, to preserve the ventral urethral skin, to detach it from the native meatus and the underlying corpora and to let it float forward as the chordee is corrected. This skin, together with the ventral skin of the glans, is then available for tubularization to form the distal portion of the neourethra. The distal end of the bladder graft is anastomosed to this tube in watertight fashion and drained to prevent stricture. Thus, no bladder mucosa is exposed, and the tendency to meatal stenosis is avoided.

During the past decade, particularly, it has become apparent that when penile skin (the available penile skin plus the doral hood) is in short supply, the neourethra should be formed from distant tissue and the foreskin saved to cover the ventral penile shaft after chordee is corrected.[12] No other available skin looks like penile skin, or has the desired innervation. Scrotal flaps may be used to surface the ventral aspect of the penile shaft proximally, but are not aesthetically pleasing unless they are perfectly centred. They remain rugated and, of course, grow hair at puberty and must be depilated if the hair growth is thick.

When foreskin is unavailable, the neourethra can be formed from full-thickness grafts of the relatively thin skin of the neck below the beard line, or from the inner arm. The harvest site scar in the neck is unsightly, however, and the arm skin is relative thick and likely to form strictures. The author has personally used free grafts of skin from the inner arm in 15 repairs; of these 15 repairs, seven developed strictures.

Bladder mucosa forms a thin graft that is vascularized rapidly and results in a neourethra that is uniform in calibre. If stenosis at the site of anastomosis to the native urethra can be prevented, a common residual problem that limits use is the tendency to stenosis where the bladder mucosa is exposed on the skin at the new meatal site. By forming the distalmost urethra from glans and penile skin, exposure of bladder mucosa and subsequent stenosis is prevented. The bladder graft can still be used to form most of the needed length of neourethra, and the penile skin and foreskin is preserved to resurface the penis.

References

1. Memmelar J. Use of bladder mucosa in a one-stage repair of hypospadias. J Urol 1947; 58: 66
2. Marshall V F, Spellman R M. Construction of urethra in hypospadias using vesical mucosal graft. J Urol 1955; 73: 335–342
3. Ehrlich R M, Reda E F, Kogle M A. Complications of bladder mucosa graft. J Urol 1989; 142: 626
4. Li Z G, Zheng Y H, Sheh Y X, Cao Y F. One-stage urethroplasty for hypospadias using a tube constructed with bladder mucosa — a new procedure. Urol Clin North Am 1981; 8: 463
5. Ransley P G, Duffy P G, Vesch I L et al. The use of bladder mucosa and combined bladder mucosa/preputial skin grafts for urethral reconstruction. J Urol 1987; 138: 1096–1098
6. King L R. Hypospadias — a one stage repair without skin graft based on a new principle: chordee is sometimes produced by skin alone. J Urol 1970; 103: 660–662
7. Coleman J W, McGovern J H, Marshall V F. The bladder mucosal graft technique for hypospadias repair. Urol Clin North Am 1981; 8: 457
8. King L R. Cutaneous chordee and its implications in hypospadias repair. Urol Clin North Am 1981; 8: 397–402

9. Van der Meulen J C. Hypospadias and cryptospadias. Br J Plast Surg 1971; 24: 101–108
10. Van der Meulen J C. Correction of hypospadias: Types I and II. Ann Plast Surg 1982; 8: 403–411
11. Byars L T. A technique for consistently satisfactory repair of hypospadias. Surg Gynecol Obstet 1955; 100: 184–190
12. Wacksman J, Sheldon C, King L R. Distal hypospadias repair. In: Webster G, Kirby R, King L, Goldwasser B (eds) Reconstructive urology. Oxford: Blackwell Scientific Publications, 1993; 749–762
13. King L R. Bladder mucosal grafts for severe hypospadias: a successful technique. J Urol 1994; 152: 2338–2340

Buccal mucosa free-grafts in complicated urethral reconstruction

3

J. R. Woodard   R. Gosalbez   J. Barone
L. M. Pérez

Introduction

In 1941, Humby was the first to report the use of both buccal and bladder mucosa free autologous grafts in the reconstruction of the male urethra.[1] Since that time a larger experience has been attained using bladder mucosa, with various reports noting complications mainly occurring at the neomeatus in 9–66% of cases.[2–5] Recently, the use of buccal mucosa in the reconstruction of the male urethra has gained significant popularity, with most publications coming from centres outside the United States.[6–9] The authors now describe their experience over a 2-year period from 1992 to 1994 with the use of buccal mucosa in complicated cases of reconstruction of the hypospadic, epispadic and duplicated male urethra.

Patients and methods

Between July 1992 and June 1994, a total of 22 reconstructive urethral procedures using autologous buccal mucosa grafts were performed on 21 male patients at the authors' institutions. Patient ages ranged from 8 months to 35 years (mean 9.6 years), with 12 patients less than 10 years of age and three less than 2 years of age. The indication for surgery was lack of sufficient penile or preputial skin in all patients with various underlying conditions (Table 3.1).

Whereas three patients (two with perineal hypospadias and penoscrotal transposition, and one with Y-duplication of the urethra) had never had previous repairs, the remaining patients had undergone between one and nine (mean 3.5) procedures previously. Of the 22 repairs, 18 entailed buccal mucosa at the neomeatus (11 onlays and 7 tubes). The length of the individual grafts ranged from 1.5 to 7.0 cm

Diagnosis	No. of patients
Previous unsuccessful hypospadias repairs	11
Perineal hypospadias with penoscrotal transposition	3
Urethral hair tuft and stone	2
Epispadias–exstrophy complex	2
Urethral stricture	2
Y-type urethral duplication	1

Table 3.1. Patient diagnosis/indications

(mean 3.9 cm) with the largest lip graft being 4.5 cm (from a 12-year-old) and the largest cheek graft being 7.0 cm (from an 18-year-old).

Surgical technique

The repair begins with correction of chordee, if present, followed by measurement of urethral defect. Whenever possible a roof strip (urethral plate) is saved so that an onlay repair can be performed. If this is not possible, a tubularized graft is necessary. Wide spatulation of the urethra is performed in preparation for anastomosis and the area is packed with moist gauze while the buccal mucosa is harvested.

The appropriate size buccal mucosa (approximately 10–20% larger than the urethral defect) is harvested using a No. 15 scalpel from either the inner surface of the lower lip or the inner cheek. Stenson's duct is avoided. Submucosal saline or 0.5% xylocaine with 1:200 000 dilution of epinephrine injection is used to allow for easier harvesting and haemostasis. Four fine corner holding sutures are placed in order to decrease handling trauma to the mucosa. Small defects do not require closure; benzocaine (Orabase) may be applied. Larger defects, especially cheek, are closed with running interlocking 4/0 chromic sutures. The graft is soaked in antibiotic saline solution and completely defatted using iris scissors. The free graft is then either used as an onlay or tubularized over an appropriately sized catheter using a running 7/0 polydioxanone suture. Following completion of the anastomosis with the native urethra, subcutaneous tissues are mobilized and brought over the graft. A urethral stent and a soft compressive dressing are placed. The patient is kept at strict bedrest for approximately 5 days. Catheters and dressings are removed 10–14 days postoperatively.

A total of 25 buccal mucosal grafts (15 lower lips and 10 cheeks) were harvested. Of those from the lip, one was used as a distal onlay anastomosed to a proximal tubularized bladder mucosa graft. Another lip mucosa was used as a distal onlay in conjunction with a proximal tubularized cheek mucosa graft. Bilateral cheek mucosae were fashioned into tubularized grafts in two patients.

Results

With a follow-up of 3–25 months (mean 10 months), morbidity has been confined primarily to strictures and fistulas (Fig. 3.1). The only other complication was a single readmission for pyelonephritis in a child with urethral duplication and bilateral vesicoureteral reflux.

No patient had any complications at the meatus. All strictures were confined to the anastomotic sites (with native urethra or bladder mucosa). In one patient both proximal and distal anastomotic strictures occurred (Fig. 3.2). Interestingly, the tubularized buccal mucosa between these anastomotic strictures was patent, as assessed by retrograde urethrogram, and quite healthy on cystoscopic examination (Fig. 3.2). When comparing the results of purely onlay grafts with those of tubularized grafts, although the former had a significantly lower rate of

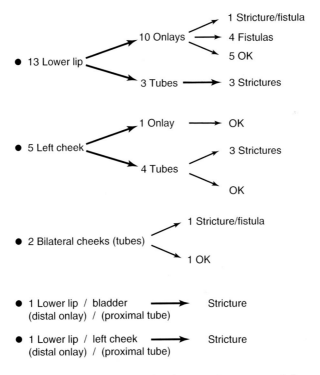

Figure 3.1. Results of buccal grafts substratified for location of tissue retrieval (lip vs cheek) and whether reconstructed as a tube or onlay.

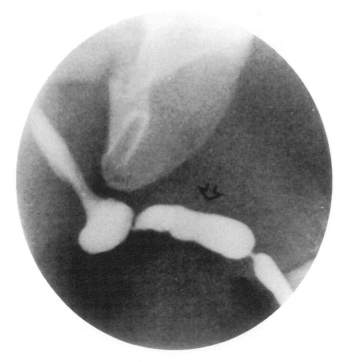

Figure 3.2. Retrograde urethrogram of 20-year-old man who had undergone urethral reconstruction with a 7.0 × 2.0 cm tubularized buccal graft over a 16 Fr catheter 2 years earlier (urethra with hair tuft and stone following scrotal inlay years earlier for penoscrotal hypospadias and penoscrotal transposition). Both proximal and distal anastomotic strictures are evident, with normal graft in between (arrow).

anastomotic stricture formation (1/11 or 9% vs 7/9 or 78%), a higher rate (although less dramatic) of fistula formation was noted (5/11 or 45% vs 1/9 or 11%). The management of these anastomotic strictures and fistulas is summarized in Table 3.2.

Tubularized grafts were used in two patients (4 and 12 years of age) undergoing reconstruction for epispadias. A severe anastomotic stricture occurred in one patient, requiring a first-stage Johanson urethroplasty. Similarly, a tubularized graft extending from the prostatomembranous region to a penoscrotal neomeatus was performed in a 15-month-old patient with Y-duplication of the urethra. This patient also developed an anastomotic stricture requiring dilatation in the operating room.

Problem	Management
Strictures (10)*	Self-dilatation (2)**
	Dilatation in OR (1)
	1st stage Johanson urethroplasty (3)†
	Thiersch–Duplay urethroplasty (1)
	Awaiting repair (3)
Fistulas (6)	Primary repair (2)
	Buccal graft (1)
	Awaiting repair (3)

*Number of patients in parentheses.
**One patient had internal urethrotomy.
†One patient had failed primary repair, and another failed internal urethrotomy.

Table 3.2. Management of anastomotic strictures and fistulas

Discussion

Autologous buccal and bladder mucosa free-grafts are alternative tissues for use in the reconstruction of the male urethra when penile or preputial skin is not available. Extragenital full-thickness skin grafts, although another option for such patients, is fraught with morbidity (primarily in the form of obliterative stricture disease).[10] The early buccal mucosa experience[6–9] has been enthusiastically received, rather as, several years ago, was the short-term follow-up of bladder mucosa.[2–5] With longer follow-up that enthusiasm decreased, mainly because of problems at the neomeatus. The authors' experience suggests that further experience and longer follow-up with buccal mucosa might see diminished enthusiasm, mainly because of anastomotic strictures. This, apparently, is not new information for those with much earlier experiences. El-Kasaby and associates reported excellent results (90% success rate) with the use of 2–4 cm buccal mucosa patch grafts for adult anterior urethral strictures.[8] In an editorial reply to their article, these authors reported that they had 'used a buccal mucosa graft for correction of crippling hypospadias since 1972 but (their) results were not as encouraging as with adult urethral strictures'.

At present, the authors are not certain as to the aetiology of the high rate of anastomotic strictures with the use of buccal mucosa grafts. Clearly, however, there is a much higher rate of such strictures in the tubularized grafts (78%) than in those used as onlays (9%). At the same time, there appears to be little tendency for neomeatal morbidity with the use of buccal grafts. The authors therefore recommend the use of buccal grafts rather than bladder grafts at the neomeatus position, and the use of buccal mucosa onlays rather than tubular configurations. In this context, one of their patients (a 15-year-old with perineal hypospadias and chordee with a previously failed procedure at early age) underwent a 10 cm tubularized bladder mucosa graft from the perineum to mid-penile shaft, and a 4 cm buccal mucosa onlay from the mid-penile region to the meatus. He too, however, developed an anastomotic stricture 4 months later between the buccal mucosa onlay and tubularized bladder mucosa graft. A Thiersch–Duplay urethroplasty was performed 2 months ago and he is awaiting further evaluation.

The occurrence of fistulas was also high, although lower for the tubular (11%) than the onlay (45%) grafts, and mostly occurred at the coronal sulcus. Although there is an inherent higher incidence of fistulas in patients with previously failed hypospadias repairs, in the authors' opinion this high rate of fistula, particularly for onlay grafts, will decrease with experience.

The high morbidity rate does not detract from the advantages of the buccal mucosa graft (i.e. minimal neomeatal problems, and ease of harvesting technique when compared with bladder mucosa). If more care is taken to prevent fistula occurrence (e.g. tunica vaginalis coverage), then the use of buccal mucosa onlays remains quite appealing. Long-term reports from other centres are awaited in order to determine whether the high rate of morbidity noted by the authors is solely technical, rather than inherent in the procedure.

References

1. Humby G. A one-stage operation for hypospadias. Br J Surg 1941; 29: 84–92
2. Hendren W H, Reda E F. Bladder mucosa graft for construction of male urethra. J Pediatr Surg 1986; 21: 189
3. Ransley P G, Duffy P G, Oesch I L, Van Oyen P, Hoover D. The use of bladder mucosa and combined bladder mucosa/preputial skin grafts for urethral reconstruction. J Urol 1987; 138: 1096–1098
4. Mollard P, Mouriquand P, Bringeon G, Bugmann P. Repair of hypospadias using a bladder bucosal graft in 76 cases. J Urol 1989; 142: 1548–1550
5. Keating M A, Cartwright P C, Duckett J W. Bladder mucosa in urethral reconstructions. J Urol 1990; 114: 827–834
6. Bürger R A, Müller S C, El-Damanhoury H et al. The buccal mucosal graft for urethral reconstruction: a preliminary report. J Urol 1992; 147: 662–664
7. Dessanti A, Rigamonti W, Merulla V et al. Autologous buccal mucosa graft for hypospadias repair: an initial report. J Urol 1992; 147: 1081–1084
8. El-Kasaby A W, Fath-Alla M, Noweir AM et al. The use of buccal mucosa patch graft in the management of anterior urethral strictures. J Urol 1993; 149: 276–278
9. Gonzalvez Pinera J, Perez Martinez A, Andujar Cairo M et al. Buccal mucosa free graft for severe hypospadias repair. Chir Pediatr 1994; 7: 48–49

10 Webster G D, Brown M W, Koefoot R B, Sihelnick S. Suboptimal results in full thickness skin graft urethroplasty using an extrapenile skin donor site. J Urol 1984; 131: 1082–1083

4

Modified transverse preputial island flap technique for severe hypospadias, combined with inverted U-shaped interscrotal flap

Y. Banya   K. Ishikura   K. Seino   J. Matsuzaka
T. Kurosawa   T. Kajikawa   T. Fujioka   T. Kubo

Introduction

One-stage repairs have recently become the mainstay in the management of hypospadias. Among numerous elegant methods introduced for the repair of hypospadias, the transverse preputial island flap technique advocated by Duckett[1-3] has proved to be an excellent one-stage operation. However, in some cases of severe hypospadias, such as penoscrotal, scrotal and perineoscrotal hypospadias, the urethral meatus is proximally located, so that the area of inner foreskin available for an island pedicle tube is not always long or wide enough to bridge the long gap to form a neourethra between the meatus and the tip of the glans. In such cases a proximal add-on neourethra can be fashioned from non-hairbearing interscrotal tissue. Glassberg[4] described a U-type of incision around the base of the urethral meatus, forming a proximal neourethra. In the authors' operation, following the Duckett transverse tube pedicle urethroplasty an inverted U-shaped incision is made around the base of the urethral meatus, forming a proximal neourethra. In addition, the operating microscope is used to facilitate suturing and anastomosis of the neourethral tube. These procedures have the advantage of decreasing the fistula rate, since the whole sutured line of the reconstructive urethral tube does not face the ventral side of the penile shaft. This chapter describes a modified transverse preputial island technique combined with the inverted U-shaped interscrotal flap method for severe hypospadias.

Technique

First, the deficit of the corpus spongiosum urethrae is identified by a sound inserted through the urethral meatus, as the sound can be seen through the ventral penile skin where the corpus spongiosum is absent. This portion of ventral penile skin is incised along the inserted sound. After a ventral incision is extended vertically 3–4 mm distal to the urethral meatus, the length of the neourethra is measured. A longer length than that of the skin portion lacking the corpus spongiosum urethrae should be selected, because the urethral meatus will have dropped back considerably from the original position by the release of chordee. Cases arise in which the neourethra becomes too long, since the meatus is proximally located. In such cases, a proximal tubular add-on neourethra should be fashioned from the non-hairbearing interscrotal skin or perineal skin. After the length of neourethra has been decided, the area of preparation of incised penile skin is outlined. A circumferential incision is made around the corona of the penis; an inverted U-shaped incision is then made around the urethral meatus along the line (Fig. 4.1). The diameter of the neourethral tube is usually accommodated by this, a 10 Fr silicone catheter easily passing through the tube.

Dissection of the penile skin is started at the dorsal side. The penile skin is carefully released just above the tunica albuginea of the penis to preserve the deep dorsal veins and the dorsal arteries during dorsal dissection. The dissection is then extended in the same plane to the

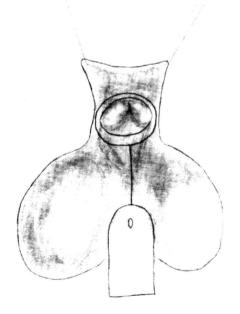

Figure 4.1. Skin incision. A circumferential incision is made around the corona of the penis following a ventral vertical incision. An inverted U-shaped incision is then made around the urethral meatus to the non-hairbearing interscrotal and perineal skin.

ventral side, while the fibrous chordee is sharply excised to straighten the penis. This excision is continued until the surface of the tunica albuginea is exposed. After urethral mobilization, the position of the penis is assessed by means of an artificial erection induced by physiological saline injected into the corpus cavernosum penis. After the chordee has been corrected completely, the inverted U-shaped incision is deepened with preparation of a pedicle and flap (Fig. 4.2).

The inverted U-shaped flap is rolled up and sutured to form the proximal neourethra. A Duckett transverse island pedicle tube is constructed from the inner foreskin as the distral neourethra (Fig. 4.3a). The sutures of the neourethra and anastomosis between the distal and proximal neourethrae are peformed under the operating microscope. The skin flap is rolled up and the subcutaneous tissues are sutured together with interrupted 6/0 polydioxanone sutures to form the neourethral tube (Fig. 4.3b).

After the distal neourethra has been formed, this tube is carefully separated from the dorsal penile skin, preserving the subcutaneous tissue. A buttonhole is bluntly formed in the centre of the pedicle. The distal neourethral tube is transposed ventrally, tunnelled distally through the glans, anastomosed to the tip of the glans, and then anastomosed proximally to the proximal neourethral tube (Fig. 4.4). In some cases, the hollow of the original meatus at the tip of the glans is vertically incised, and then the subcutaneous tissue is dissected into a cylindrical shape to

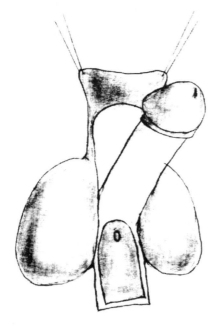

Figure 4.2. Skin dissection and chordee release. Dissection of the penile skin is started at the dorsal side. The penile skin is carefully released just above the tunica albuginea of the penis. The dissection is then extended in the same plane to the ventral side, while the fibrous chordee is sharply excised to straighten the penis. An inverted U-shaped incision is deepened with preparation of pedicle and flap.

a

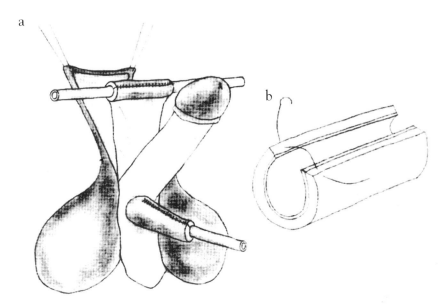

b

Figure 4.3. (a) The proximal neourethra and distal neourethra are fashioned. An inverted U-shaped flap is rolled up and sutured to form the proximal neourethra. A Duckett transverse island pedicle tube is constructed from the inner foreskin as the distal neourethra. (b) The sutures of the neourethra and anastomosis between the distal and proximal neourethrae are inserted under the operating microscope. The skin flap is rolled up and the subcutaneous sutured tissues are sutured together with interrupted 6/0 polydioxanone sutures to form the neourethral tube.

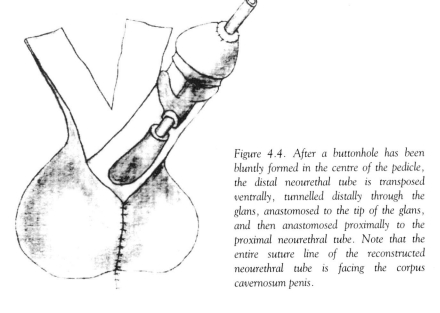

Figure 4.4. After a buttonhole has been bluntly formed in the centre of the pedicle, the distal neourethal tube is transposed ventrally, tunnelled distally through the glans, anastomosed to the tip of the glans, and then anastomosed proximally to the proximal neourethral tube. Note that the entire suture line of the reconstructed neourethral tube is facing the corpus cavernosum penis.

protect the inserted distal neourethral tube from compression. When the proximal and distal tubes have been anastomosed, the excess portion of the neourethral tube is cut off and the tube is sutured. This incision is easily performed after the meatoplasty. If the proximal neourethral tube is long enough, it should be sutured to the corpus cavernosum penis.

The reconstructed neourethral tube is completely covered by the subcutaneous tissue. The neourethral tube must be further covered by the dartos or the tunica vaginalis. After the scrotum has been sutured, Byar's flaps are fashioned and the skin flaps are brought together vertically into the midline or are interdigitated. After the operation, a suprapubic catheter is always used without a urethral catheter. A pressure dressing is applied and left in place for 4 days. To prevent the meatus drying out, gentamycin sulfate ointment was applied to the tip of the glans. The catheter is removed 10–14 days after the operation, and micturition is started.

Results

From 1989 to 1994, this procedure was used in 18 cases of severe hypospadias, with a mean follow-up period of 2 years (range 8 months to 6 years). Fistula complicated two early cases (11.1%); these were repaired 6 months later. No other complication has been noted. Thus, 16 out of 18 boys obtained satisfactory cosmetic and functional results with a single operation (Table 4.1).

Discussion

The one-stage repair for severe hypospadias using an operating microscope gives a high operative success rate, as the genital skin is used as a graft to form a urethral tube with a total sutured line that does not face the ventral side of the penile shaft. Patients with severe hypospadias usually have shiny, non-hairbearing skin lying in the midline between each hemiscrotum distal to the hypospadiac meatus. In such cases Duckett has advocated using this skin to form the proximal neourethra.[2] Glassberg has also advocated forming a similar proximal neourethra in cases of penoscrotal hypospadias.[4] However, the suture line of the U-type skin flap described by Duckett[2] and by Glassberg[4] faces the ventral side of the penile shaft. In their operation procedure, it is difficult to release chordee, because the distal portion of the U-type skin flap is located on the chordee. In contrast, the authors' inverted U-shaped skin flap enables chordee to be released completely. In addition, the incidence of fistula formation, which is the most frequent complication of urethroplasty, is markedly reduced in the procedure described here. In summary, the

Patient no.	Age (years)	Preoperative hypospadias	Postoperative complications
1	5	Penoscrotal	Fistula
2	2	Scrotal	–
3	3	Penoscrotal	Fistula
4	2	Perineal*	–
5	2	Perineal**	–
6	2	Perineal**	–
7	2	Penoscrotal	–
8	3	Penoscrotal	–
9	5	Scrotal**	–
10	2	Scrotal	––
11	6	Penoscrotal	–
12	2	Penoscrotal†	–
13	2	Scrotal*	–
14	2	Penoscrotal	–
15	2	Scrotal*	–
16	2	Penoscrotal*	–
17	2	Penoscrotal*	–
18	2	Penoscrotal	–

*Bifid scrotum.
**Transposition of the penis and scrotum.
†Abdominal testis on both sides.

Table 4.1. Preoperative and postoperative clinical findings in 18 cases of hypospadias

important points of this procedure are as follows: (1) fashioning of an inverted U-shaped flap; (2) use of an operating microscope; (3) subcutaneous suturing only; (4) positioning of the suture line to face the corpus cavernosum penis; (5) covering of the dartos; (6) use of a suprapubic catheter, and (7) keeping the meatus moist. This procedure is recommended in cases of severe hypospadias as the first-choice repair operation allowing the surgeon to bridge large gaps in a one-stage procedure.

References

1. Duckett J W. Transverse preputial island flap technique for repair of severe hypospadias. Urol Clin North Am 1980; 7: 423–430
2. Duckett J W. Hypospadias. In: Walsh P C, Gittes R F, Perlmutter A D, Stamy T A (eds) Campbell's Urology, 5th ed. Philadelphia: Saunders, 1986: 1969–1999

3. Duckett J W. Hypospadias. In: Walsh P C, Retik A B, Stamy T A, Vaughan E D (eds) Campbell's Urology, 6th ed. Philadephia: Saunders, 1992: 1893–1919
4. Glassberg K I. Augmented Duckett repair for severe hypospadias. J Urol 1987; 138: 380–381

One-stage urethroplasty with double blood supply method: a new procedure for hypospadias repair

5

E. Higashihara

Introduction

Of the numerous ingenious methods introduced to repair hypospadias, one-stage correction methods tend to be the most widely accepted. The innovation of one-stage repair dates back to 1900, when Russell described a procedure using a urethral tube constructed from the ventral foreskin of the penis.[1] Broadbent et al.[2] described one of the pioneering works of one-stage repair of hypospadias using a full-thickness oblique strip of preputial foreskin, and Asopa et al.[3] devised a one-stage repair using a foreskin flap tube. These methods are innovative, but the skin design is asymmetrical, hence potentially distorting the penis.

Duckett[4,5] developed the transverse preputial island flap (TPIF) and glans channel method as a modification of the Hodgson III[6] and Asopa[3] procedures. Duckett[7] then reported a double-faced preputial island flap (DPIF) method as a combined modification of his own transverse preputial island flap method and the preputial island flap technique reported by Standoli.[8] According to the original description, they mobilized the neourethra from the dorsum to the ventrum of the penis by a lateral route,[7,8] and later through a buttonhole opening at the centre of the pedicle. In this method, outer preputial skin served as a skin cover for the neourethra, which was constructed from inner preputial foreskin. This skin cover was expected to reduce the incidence of urethral fistulas because the sutured side of the neourethra faced the penis and the ventral side of the neourethra was covered with an outer plate of foreskin. However, one of the crucial points in reducing postoperative fistula formation is an adequate blood supply to the neourethra and covering skin. The major role of the blood supply is shown by the frequent complication rate in urethroplasty using free skin grafts.[9] In

43

preputial island flap methods, vascularity to the new urethral tube is supplied mainly from the superficial dorsal arteries of the penis and may be inadequate. In addition, the transversely formed urethra must be rotated vertically after transposition of an island flap to the ventrum, and the rotation of the pedicle may impair blood flow to the island flap.

Koyanagi et al. described a one-stage urethroplasty using a parameatal foreskin flap,[10,11] and demonstrated an adequate blood supply to this extended skin flap.[12] In this method, vascularity to the neourethra is maintained via the base of the parameatal foreskin flap.

On the basis of the present author's experience with Asopa's technique[13] and preputial island flap methods,[14] a new technique has been developed that provides a double blood supply to the neourethra both from superficial dorsal vessels of the penis and from the base of parameatal foreskin flaps.[15] The method does not require rotation of the pedicle.

Technique

The method of repair described in this chapter is applicable to those patients with mild to severe hypospadias. Two skin incisions are made. First, a circumferential incision is made 2–3 mm proximal to the corona, but this does not include the meatus. The dissection is carried out to free the dorsal penile skin and prepuce in the avascular plane that exists between the superficial fascia of the penis and Buck's fascia. This plane is generally easily identified at the 2 and 10 o'clock positions and is the same plane as that dissected in the island flap method.[4,5,7] The superficial dorsal veins and arteries of the penis attach to the skin side, while the deep dorsal vessels remain on the penile side.[16] When dissection is extended to the lateral and ventral aspects along this plane, chordee tissue is found around Buck's fascia. Extensive excision of the area of chordee is necessary around the urethra and Buck's fascia. The urethra is dissected from the penile shaft and mobilization of the urethra results in transposition of the meatus back to the penoscrotal junction or even to the scrotum. Adequacy of the chordectomy is tested by an artificial erection technique. The penile shaft becomes denuded when this step is completed (Fig. 5.1).

When chordectomy is completed, a second skin incision is outlined using a centimetre rule and a marking pencil. The second skin incision is proximal to the first one and includes the meatus. While the foreskin is extended to cover the glans of the penis, the dorsal and lateral side of the foreskin is marked semicircumferentially approximately 5 mm distal to the underlying corona. On the ventral side of the penis, the right and left lines of the skin incision are extended proximally to include the meatus and form the parameatal skin flap. The parameatal skin flap is about

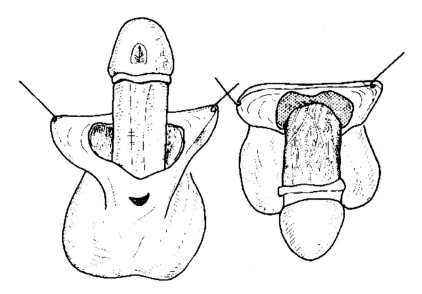

Figure 5.1. The skin incision is circumferential and 2–3 mm proximal to the corona. The deep dorsal veins remain on the penile side during dorsal dissection. During extension of this plane to the ventral side, chordee tissue is found around Buck's fascia.

10–12 mm wide, depending on the size of the neourethra. The entire second incision must be superficial and avoid cutting the subcutaneous tissue, thus permitting vascularity of the skin flap from a wide area of subcutaneous tissue (Fig. 5.2).

A plane is developed between the dorsal penile skin and its underlying vascular pedicle. This dissection plane is the same as that created for the pedicle of the new urethra in the island flap method.[5] The pedicle includes the superficial penile fascia and the superficial dorsal veins of the penis and is attached to the skin flap used for the neourethra. Care must be taken during this dissection not to injure the blood vessels of the pedicle. Dissection is continued approximately 15–20 mm proximal to the edge of the dorsal skin and a buttonhole is made in the base of the pedicle to transpose the foreskin to the ventrum (Figs 5.2 and 5.3).

The skin aperture that originally attached to the corona is closed with interrupted 7/0 polydioxanone sutures. An 8 or 10 Fr stent is passed into the bladder and the neourethra is created around the stent with interrupted 7/0 polydioxanone sutures using a threefold magnification operating microscope. Meticulous care is taken in joining each vascular layer during suturing of the neourethra and to avoid inversion of the epithelial surfaces (Fig. 5.4). Occasionally, the foreskin flap for the neourethra becomes redundant and forms a recess at the level above the

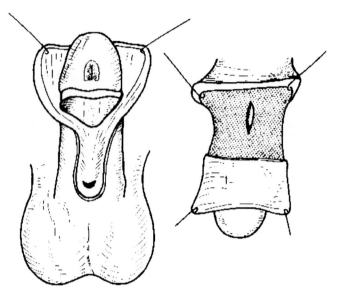

Figure 5.2. When chordectomy is completed, a second skin incision is made. The dorsal foreskin is incised circumferentially and the incision is extended to include the meatus on the ventrum. Dissection is carried out between the dorsal penile skin and the underlying vasular pedicle.

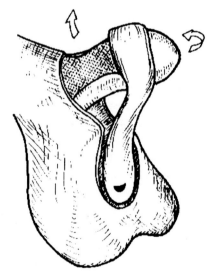

Figure 5.3. A buttonhole is made in the base of the pedicle to transpose the dorsal foreskin to the ventrum.

closed aperture. This foreskin recess is not a problem when creating the neourethra, but when the neourethra is longer than necessary, as in distal hypospadias, the urethral tip might be made alternatively at the bottom of the recess. In this case, the ventral portion of the distal neourethra is

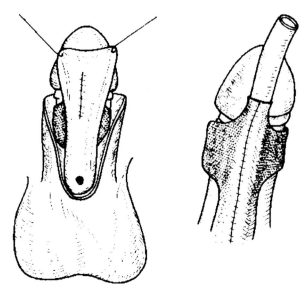

Figure 5.4. A skin aperture, the edge of which was originally attached to the corona, is closed and a neourethra is created with 7/0 polydioxanone around a stent.

formed by a reflected preputial outer plate. An aperture is made at the skin reflection to create a new meatus. In either case, the urethra is made from both dorsal and parameatal foreskin and is usually sufficiently long, even in severe hypospadias. Anastomosis of the neourethra to the original urethra is not necessary because of the continuity of the neourethra with the original meatus.

The glans channel is then created and the distal portion of the neourethra is delivered through the channel. The neourethra is pulled out so that no redundant tissue remains and the excess tip of the neourethra is excised. Five or six interrupted polydioxanone sutures (6/0) are used to secure the edge of the glandular channel to the edge of the neourethra. This part of the technique is essentially similar to that in the TPIF method.[5] An 8 or 10 Fr polyethylene feeding tube is placed through the neourethra into the bladder as a stent and indwelling catheter. The catheter is fixed to the glans with a 4/0 nylon suture. Cystostomy is not usually performed.

The dorsal penile skin is approximated to the corona in a manner similar to circumcision. The flaps of penile skin are brought around to the ventrum so that closure can be achieved in a symmetrical fashion. Suturing is performed with interrupted 6/0 polydioxanone sutures. Some of the subcutaneous tissue from the penile skin flaps may be brought together to cover the urethral sutures (Fig. 5.5).

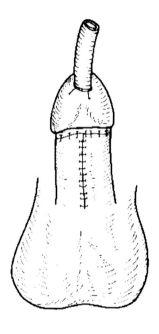

Figure 5.5. A glans channel is made and the distal portion of the neourethra is passed through the channel. The skin is approximated as shown here.

Results

Initially, Asopa's method was used in 15 patients. Eight patients developed urethral fistulas and one had a urethral stricture; each of these complications was subsequently corrected with a single operation. However, penile distortion occurred in three patients due to the asymmetrical rotation of the foreskin flap to the ventrum. To avoid penile distortion, TPIF and DPIF techniques were then adopted in four and five patients, respectively. There was no postoperative penile deformity but fistula formation was encountered in eight patients; correction of these fistulas required an average of 2.8 operations.

The double blood supply method was developed and applied to the next seven patients. The types of hypospadias were coronal (one), proximal penile (four), penoscrotal (one) and perineal (one). The patient with perineal hypospadias had a dysplastic male syndrome. There was no postoperative distortion or urethral stricture. Urethral fistulas developed in three patients and were subsequently corrected with a single operation. Reconstruction of the glandular urethra was successful in seven patients.

There was less frequent fistula formation after the double blood supply procedure than after the island flap procedure and penile distortion was avoided using this new technique.

Discussion

Two-stage surgery has a number of shortcomings compared with one-stage urethroplasty. First, there is psychological trauma for young patients, because the meatus may be as far back as the perineum after the first stage of surgery, which forces a boy to void in a sitting position. Second, repeated surgery is more expensive and time-consuming than a single operation. In addition, repeated surgery at the same site leads to marked fibrosis and tends to give rise to more frequent fistulas and strictures. Third, urethral skin often comprises penile proximal skin because it is practically impossible to exclude the penile skin from the urethra at the second operation. Encompassing penile skin in the urethra produces intraurethral hairs later. Fourth, the meatus cannot be created at the tip of the glans in most two-stage urethroplasties.

One-stage urethroplasty resolves these disadvantages of two-stage surgery. The goals that must be achieved in one-stage procedures include (a) complete release of chordee, (b) the creation of a neourethra without resultant urethral fistula, stricture or diverticulum, (c) positioning of the meatus at the apex of the glans and (d) coverage of the penis with skin that is pliable, elastic and symmetrical.

In Asopa's method and the island flap technique, complete removal of chordee is possible and there is no penile kinking postoperatively when chordectomy is performed appropriately. In the double blood supply method, the procedure to release chordee is the same as that in those methods and there has been no case of incomplete chordectomy. The most frequent problem of urethroplasty is fistula formation. Although the fistula rate was high in the author's series using TPIF and DPIF methods compared with that in the reports of Duckett,[4,5] a relatively high fistula formation rate was reported in the TPIF procedure by others.[17] In the author's experience, there was less frequent fistula formation after Asopa's method had been used than after either the TPIF or DPIF methods. A fistula is probably formed when the blood supply to the neourethra is inadequate. The island flap has the advantage of covering the penis cosmetically, but it may compromise the blood supply to the neourethra. The double blood supply method was developed to ensure that sufficient blood is supplied to the neourethra while maintaining the advantage of the island flap method, i.e. creating the meatus at the apex of the glans and coverage of the penis with skin that is cosmetic, symmetrical and non-hairbearing. In the double blood supply method, the neourethra is fed not only from the same vascular sources as those in the island flap procedure but also from the parameatal skin flap. This enhancement of blood supply seems to contribute to improving the results of urethroplasty.

In conclusion, the use of a double blood supply method to create the neourethra maintains excellent vascularity, thereby ensuring wound healing, which is the most critical aspect of this type of surgery. Skin coverage is natural and symmetrical, resulting in a good cosmetic appearance.

References

1. Russell R H. Operation for severe hypospadias. Br Med J 1900; 2: 1432–1435
2. Broadbent T R, Woolf R B, Toksu E. Hypospadias, one-stage repair. Plast Recontr Surg 1961; 25: 154–159
3. Asopa H S, Elhence I P, Atri S P, Bansal N K. One stage correction of hypospadias using a foreskin tube. A preliminary report. Int Surg 1971; 55: 435–440
4. Duckett J W Jr. Transverse preputial island flap technique for repair of severe hypospadias. Urol Clin North Am 1980; 7: 423–430
5. Duckett J W Jr. The island flap technique for hypospadias repair. Urol Clin North Am 1981; 8: 503–519
6. Hodgson N B. Hypospadias. In: Glenn G F, Boyce W H (eds) Urologic Surgery, 2nd ed. Hagerstown: Harper and Row, 1975: 656–667
7. Duckett J W. Hypospadias. In: Walsh P C, Gittes R F, Perlmutter A D, Stamey T A, (eds). Cambell's Urology, 5th ed. Philadelphia: Saunders, 1986: 1969–1999
8. Standoli L. One-stage repair of hypospadias: preputial island flap technique. Ann Plast Surg 1982; 9: 81–88
9. Valla J S, Takvorian P H, Dodat H *et al*. Single-stage correction of posterior hypospadias (178 cases). Comparison of three techniques: free skin graft, free bladder mucosal graft, transverse pedicle preputial graft. Eur J Pediatr Surg 1991; 1: 287–290
10. Koyanagi T, Matsuno T, Nonomura K *et al*. Complete repair of severe penoscrotal hypospadias in 1 stage: experience with urethral mobilization, wing flap-flipping urethroplasty and granulomeatoplasty. J Urol 1983; 130: 1150–1154
11. Koyanagi T, Nonomura K, Gotoh T *et al*. One-stage repair of perineal hypospadias and scrotal transposition. Eur Urol 1984; 10: 364–367
12. Nonomura K, Koyanagi T, Imanaka K, Asano Y. Measurement of blood flow in the parameatal foreskin flap for urethroplasty in hypospadias repair. Eur Urol 1992; 21: 155–159
13. Higashihara E, Kakizawa Y. One-stage urethroplasty — a modification of Asopa's method. J Jpn Soc Pediatr Surg 1984; 20: 341–348 (in Japanese)
14. Higashihara E, Minowada S. One stage urethroplasty using preputial inner skin. Urol Surg 1991; 4: 37–42 (in Japanese)
15. Higashihara E. Urinary tract anomaly. In: Ishida M, Nakajoy T, Tsuchida Y (eds) Pediatric surgery, new edition. Tokyo: Shindan To Chiryousha, 1994: 317–323 (in Japanese)
16. Hinman F Jr. Penis and male urethra. In: Atlas of urosurgical anatomy. Philadelphia: Saunders, 1993: 417–470
17. Dewan P A, Dinneen M D, Winkle D *et al*. Hypospadias: Duckett pedicle tube urethroplasty. Eur Urol 1991; 20: 39–42

Repair of meatal retraction: a modified onlay island flap technique

6

K. Watanabe   A. Ogawa

Introduction

Persistent hypospadias with meatal retraction is a sequel of unsuccessful hypospadias repair. Although a retracted meatus remaining within the glans seldom causes clinical problems,[1] one that has regressed beyond the corona causes significant spraying or deflection of the urinary stream and requires revision. For these patients, meatal-based flap urethroplasty has been recommended.[2-4] However, some patients have insufficient ventral penile skin for construction of a meatal-based flap. The authors have modified the onlay island flap procedure[5] and applied it to such patients.

Surgical technique

Parallel skin incisions approximately 7–11 mm apart are made on both sides of the urethral plate, with a narrowed span at the tip of the glans (Fig. 6.1a). One of these incisions is extended longitudinally along the previously constructed neourethra. Subcoronal skin incisions are made on both sides and a semicircumferential incision is made 1–2 mm proximal to the retracted meatus. The ventral skin is separated from the previously constructed neourethra, and the lateral skin and dartos fascia are dissected from the shaft (Fig. 6.1b). A vertical, rectangular flap with a subcutaneous pedicle is obtained from the dissected lateral skin (Fig. 6.1c). The flap is approximately 9–13 mm wide and approximately 2 mm longer than the urethral plate. After the glans wings are dissected laterally, the flap is brought over on to the urethral plate and is closed with running sutures on both sides (Fig. 6.1d). The subcutaneous pedicle covers the suture lines and is fixed to the tunica albuginea to avoid fistula formation (Fig. 6.1e). The glans wings are wrapped over the glanular urethra with deep and epithelial sutures (Fig. 6.1f, g). A urethral indwelling catheter is left in place for 6 days.

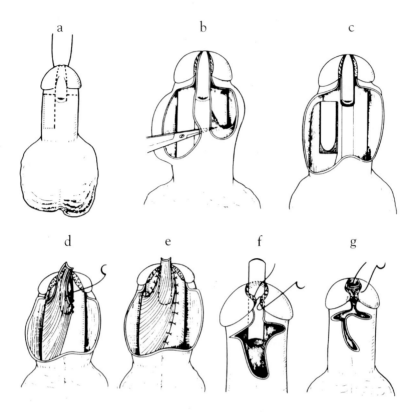

Figure 6.1. Modified onlay island flap technique for correction of meatal retraction. (a) Dashed lines mark skin incisions; dotted line indicates the epithelial incision. (b) The ventral skin is separated from the previously constructed neourethra. Separation is started from the base of the shaft to avoid injury to the neourethra. Dotted line indicates epithelial incision. (c) Rectangular skin with abundant subcutaneous tissue is obtained from the lateral skin. The flap edge is trimmed (hatched area) to fit it to the urethral plate and to ensure flap vascularization. (d) The flap is brought over on to the urethral plate and closed with running sutures on both sides. (e) The pedicle covers the suture lines. (f) The deep tissues of the glans wings are approximated with 5/0 or 6/0 polydioxanone sutures over a 16–24 Fr sound to avoid constricting the glanular urethra. (g) The flap tip is sutured to the epithelial layer of the glans with 5/0 or 6/0 polydioxanone sutures.

Results

From December 1990 the authors applied this technique to seven patients (two adults and five children), ranging in age from 4 to 29 years (mean age 12 years). Each patient had undergone between two and five repair operations. The latest procedure they had undergone was the King procedure (four patients), the Denis Browne (one), the Mathieu (one) and the Mustarde (one). Follow-up ranged from 13 to 40 months (mean 23 months). Postoperative complications requiring revision occurred in three patients. Of these, one developed penile rotation and slight meatal retraction. The penile rotation was corrected by a simple skin incision and the meatal retraction by the MAGPI procedure.[6] Another patient developed meatal stenosis, which was successfully treated by a simple incision. The third patient developed severe meatal stenosis due to dense intraglanular fibrosis. After the fibrosis had been excised, a buccal mucosa flap[7] was used to reconstruct a new glanular urethra. Further stenosis at the mucosal anastomosis required yet another revision.

Discussion

A skin flap with a subcutaneous pedicle obtained from the penile skin has been used for repair of meatal stenosis or urethral stricture.[8,9] However, its application to meatal retraction has not been reported. The onlay island flap procedure using a vascularized island flap of tissue from the inner prepuce was initially designed for mid or distal penile hypospadias,[5] and has been applied to proximal hypospadias.[10] Postoperative meatal retraction differs from primary distal hypospadias in that the retraction accompanies not an abundance of preputial skin but a superfluity of penile skin. It seems reasonable, therefore, to use this penile skin to repair meatal retraction.

On the basis of an anatomical study, Hinman[11] has emphasized that when an inner preputial island flap is created, the outer preputial skin used as the ventral cover will become ischaemic. Duckett has stated that the outer extents of the inner preputial island flap are not well vascularized and are excised during the skin cover phase.[4] Although the authors did not discard any penile skin at operation, no patients developed skin necrosis. As the superfluous penile skin has thicker subcutaneous tissue than the prepuce, the skin would be still well vascularized after an island flap has been constructed. Furthermore, none of the authors' patients developed necrosis of the neourethra, despite the fact that their penile skin had been incised several times previously and the adequacy of the blood supply for the neourethra had been unpredictable. This result suggests that the previously transferred penile skin has been revascularized sufficiently from every direction.

The cause of postoperative penile rotation appears to be a short subcutaneous pedicle. If the rotation had been noted during operation, it would have been corrected by elongating the pedicle or rearranging the penile skin. Postoperative meatal stenosis probably resulted from blood supply to the pedicle being compromised by tight glans closure. The patient, who had undergone hypospadias repair with a glans splitting technique and who possessed a small, flat glans, postoperatively developed dense intraglanular fibrosis. When the glans has an inadequate blood supply, therefore, especially in patients with small, flat glans, the attempt to position a neomeatus at the glans tip may be unsuccessful.

Postoperative meatal retraction can be corrected by any technique for distal hypospadias (e.g. the MAGPI procedure, the Mathieu, the Mustarde), if that technique is appropriate to the meatal position and skin conditions. In the authors' opinion this modified onlay island flap procedure may be useful in correcting meatal retraction in the presence of superfluous lateral penile skin.

References

1. Hastie K J, Deshpande S S, Moisey C U. Long-term follow-up of the MAGPI operation for distal hypospadias. Br J Urol 1989; 63: 320–322
2. Teague J L, Roth D R, Gonzales E T. Repair of hypospadias complications using the meatal based flap urethroplasty. J Urol 1994; 151: 470–472
3. Koff S A, Brinkmann J, Ulrich J, Deighton D. Extensive mobilization of the urethral plate and urethra for repair of hypospadias: the modified Barcat technique. J Urol 1994; 151: 466–469
4. Duckett J W. Hypospadias. In: Walsh P C, Retik A B, Stamey T A, Vaughan E D Jr (eds) Campbell's Urology, 6th ed. Philadelphia: Saunders, 1992: 1893–1916
5. Elder J S, Duckett J W, Snyder H M. Onlay island flap in the repair of mid and distal penile hypospadias without chordee. J Urol 1987; 138: 376–379
6. Duckett J W, Snyder H M. Meatal advancement and glanuloplasty hypospadias repair after 1000 cases: avoidance of meatal stenosis and regression. J Urol 1992; 147: 665–669
7. Dessanti A, Rigamonti W, Merulia V et al. Autologous buccal mucosa graft for hypospadias repair: an initial report. J Urol 1992; 147: 1081–1084
8. Palmer J M, Bishai M B. Island pedicle graft in the correction of urethral meatal stenosis following hypospadias repair. J Urol 1986; 135: 1227–1228
9. Turner-Warwick R. The use of pedicle grafts in the repair of urinary tract fistulae. Br J Urol 1972; 44: 644–656
10. Baskin L S, Duckett J W, Ueoka K et al. Changing concepts of hypospadias curvature lead to more onlay island flap procedures. J Urol 1994; 151: 191–196
11. Hinman F Jr. The blood supply to preputial island flaps. J Urol 1992; 145: 1232–1235

Mathieu hypospadias repair: postoperative care

7

D. C. S. Gough   A. Dickson   T. Tsang

Introduction

The Mathieu repair, or 'flip-flap' operation, is now a very common procedure for distal hypospadias repair when no chordee is present, with few surgical complications. Reoperation is usually necessary if the patient develops a fistula or meatal stenosis.

There is little agreement in the literature as to whether the operation should be performed with the patient as a day patient without urethral drainage, or whether the patient should be in hospital with urethral drainage for 2–10 days. The aim of the authors was to assess, in a prospective randomized study, whether there was any difference in the incidence of complications if patients received either 2 or 5 days of silastic foam dressing and urinary drainage following the Mathieu repair.

Patients and methods

Ninety-two patients of median age 1.9 years (range 0.3–11 years) were randomized to have either 2 days (group A; n=43) or 5 days (group B; n=49) of treatment with silastic foam dressing following Mathieu repair (Fig. 7.1). Urinary diversion with either suprapubic or urethral catheterization was maintained until the dressing had been removed. Six patients from group B were excluded because of early removal of dressing due to excessive wetting (five) and catheter blockage (one). Eighty-five patients were, therefore, followed up for a median period of 1.5 months (range 0.3–24 months).

Results

Complications were classified as either breakdown of the anastomosis, healing with urethral fistula, or subsequent meatal stenosis. The incidence of these complications is shown in Table 7.1.

Hospital stay was significantly shorter in group A (median 4 days, range 2–6 days) than in group B (median 7 days, range 5–9 days)

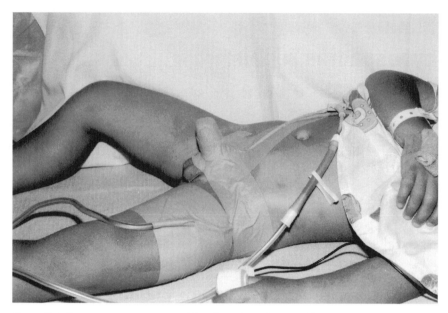

Figure 7.1. Postoperative appearance of the silastic foam dressing following Mathieu repair, with urethral and suprapubic catheters.

Complications	No. of patients	
	Group A (n=43)	Group B (n=42)
Breakdown of flap	2 (4.6)*	—
Urethral fistula	—	1 (2.4)
Meatal stenosis	—	1 (2.4)
Total	2 (4.6)	2 (4.8)

*Percentages in parentheses.

Table 7.1. Incidence of complications in patients receiving 2 days (group A) or 5 days (group B) of treatment with silastic foam dressing following Mathieu hypospadias repair

(p=0.0001; Mann–Whitney U-test, with a p-value ≤ 0.05 being regarded as statistically significant).

Comment

In his original description of this surgical procedure, Mathieu did not advocate urinary drainage, but neither did he report his complication rate. Although the Mathieu procedure is now a commonly performed operation, there have been suggestions that bladder drainage is unnecessary after surgery.[1] In their study of 21 children, Wheeler et al. used bladder drainage with a dripping stent, or no bladder drainage and no dressing, with the patient being discharged the same day. Their suggestion was that no stenting allowed early discharge and the complication rate was relatively small; however, more detailed analysis of their figures reveals that there were three patients who developed fistula and, therefore, a complication rate requiring reoperation of nearly 15%.[1] This seems a little excessive, compared with other reports of large groups of patients where a reoperation rate of 3.4% is more likely.[2] A reoperation rate for complications in about 5% of patients seems to be a much more generally accepted figure for this procedure, although others have reported reoperation rates of 8 and 11%.[3,4]

In regularly auditing their own hypospadias surgery, the authors would normally expect to see a complication rate of fistula or stenosis in less than 5% of those patients undergoing surgery for hypospadias without chordee. It was not certain, however, whether their surgical technique or the postoperative care could be modified to reduce this complication rate and allow early postoperative discharge. There is considerable pressure in health care systems for early discharge. Provided that this is not accompanied by an increased level of complications, this would seem to be a laudable objective.

A review of the literature showed a recommendation of postoperative catheter drainage of anything between 2 and 10 days,[5-7] without any controlled studies to determine which recommendations were based on scientific rather than subjective opinion. This study, therefore, set out to determine whether the complication rate and reoperation rate of the Mathieu repair was increased with early discharge from hospital. It was shown conclusively that this was not the case and that 2 days of silastic foam dressing and urinary drainage were all that was necessary to keep patients comfortable and minimize postoperative complications.

The authors have not been impressed by the concept of day case repair because of the high incidence of immediate dysuria, as reported by others, and the apparent increase in late surgical complications.[1] Although the overall cost of treatment may be minimized by day case surgery, the published incidence of long-term complications is such that the authors continue to recommend that patients are drained by catheter for 48 h, with silastic foam dressing. Because many of these patients travel for a considerable distance for surgical treatment, it is usually ensured that they are passing urine comfortably and pain free before discharge, which accounts for the length of stay in group A (a median of 4 days). With the increasing use of early repair in the first year of life this is no longer a problem and the authors are much happier to discharge patients early following removal of their dressing and stent.

Conclusions

Mathieu repair is a safe and reliable procedure for the correction of distal hypospadias without chordee. A surgical complication rate of less than 5% would seem acceptable in this procedure and can be achieved with limited hospital stay and 2 days postoperative urinary drainage and foam dressing. Longer periods of urinary drainage are not associated with any apparent benefit to the patient, and the published results of day case repair without drainage suggests that an increased complication rate may accompany this form of postoperative care.

References

1. Wheeler R A, Malone P S, Griffiths D M, Burge D M. The Mathieu operation. Is a urethral stent mandatory? Br J Urol 1993; 71: 492–495
2. Belloli G. The Mathieu Righini technique for mid-distal hypospadias repair. Pediatr Surg Int 1994; 9: 99–102
3. Gonzales E T Jr, Veeraraghavan K A, Delaune J. The management of distal hypospadias with meatal based vascularized flaps. J Urol 1983; 129: 119–120
4. Dolatzas T, Chiotopoulous D, Antipas S et al.. Hypospadias in children — review of 250 cases. Pediatr Surg Int 1994; 9: 383–386
5. Wacksman J. Modification of the one stage flip-flap procedure for repair of distal penile hypospadias. Urol Clin North Am 1981; 8: 527
6. Kim S H, Hendren W H. Repair of mild hypospadias. J Pediatr Surg 1981; 16: 806–811
7. Man D W K, Vordermark J S, Ransley P G. Experience with single stage hypospadias reconstruction. J Pediatr Surg 1986; 21: 338–341

Congenital penile curvature in childhood

8

D. Yachia

Introduction

In research conducted during 1990 to assess the incidence of congenital penile curvature it was found that 0.6% of male neonates have some degree of penile curvature.[1]

With increasing awareness, among the paediatricians and parents, of this penile deformity, more and more children are being referred for consultation, opinion and treatment.

Patients and methods

After obtaining very satisfactory results with a simple corporoplasty technique modified for straightening penile curvatures,[2] over a 3-year period from May 1991 to April 1994 the author has started to treat penile curvature in children. The technique being used is based on the Heineke–Mikulicz principle, shortening the convex part of the corpora cavernosa by closing horizontally the longitudinal incisions made in the tunica albuginea.

In order to evaluate the degree of curvature, the author recommends that the child's parents photograph the penis during erection (Fig. 8.1). If this is not possible, the deformity can be seen on examination. Penile tumescence can be induced by manually pressing the crura of the corpora cavernosa from the perineum, or by using a small vacuum device developed by the author[1,3] (Fig. 8.2).

From 1 May 1991 to 30 April 1994, 19 children with congenital penile curvature and 14 children with hypospadias with residual curvature after complete excision of the chordee have been treated using the technique described below.

Surgical technique

The penis is degloved by a circumcisional incision about 5–8 mm from the coronal sulcus. If the child has not been circumcized, a cirumcision is performed to prevent severe postoperative oedema of the prepuce. During

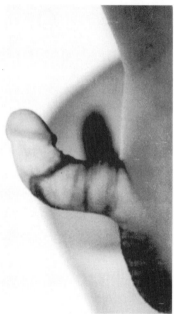

Figure 8.1. Severe dorsal penile curvature in a 4-year-old child, as seen in a photograph taken by the parents.

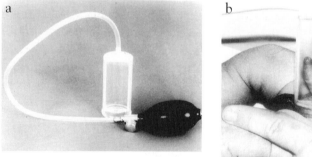
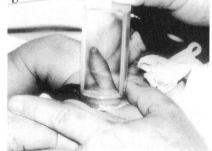

Figure 8.2. (a) Miniaturized vacuum device designed by the author to create an artificial erection for outpatient assessment of penile curvature. (b) Lateral penile curvature in a neonate as seen during an artificial erection induced by negative pressure created in the chamber of the device.

this degloving, great care should be taken not to injure the corpus spongiosum and the neurovascular bundle. However, the depth of the degloving should reach the Buck's fascia.

After retracting the penile skin downwards a tourniquet is applied at the base of the penis and an artificial erection is created by injecting saline into one of the corpora cavernosa using a thin butterfly needle. Allis clamps are then applied to the most convex parts of the corpora, taking bites of 10 mm or less in length in order to preview the result of the straightening. These bites are helpful in determining the exact site and number of incisions necessary to correct the curvature. In cases of dorsal curvature the Allis clamps are applied to both sides of the corpus spongiosum; in ventral curvatures they are applied to both sides of the neurovascular bundle and in lateral curvature to the most convex part of the contralateral corpus cavernosum. After the clamps have been removed, a longitudinal incision, tangential to the erectile tissues, is made between the marks left by the clamps on the tunica albuginea. This incision is sutured transversally using 4/0 or 5/0 Maxon sutures. The resulting bulges at the ends of the suture line are smoothed by burying sutures using the same material. The alignment and watertightness of the closure are monitored by repeating the artificial erection. The penile skin is then pulled to its normal position after removal of the tourniquet and meticulous haemostasis. Approximation of the edges is done using 5/0 Dexon sutures. At the end of the procedure a penile block is performed to ease postoperative pain. The bladder is then filled and a suprapubic cystostomy tube is positioned; the penis is dressed using a Telfa type non-adhesive dressing and, if the penis is long enough, a 5 cm wide elastic bandage is applied around it to prevent haematoma and oedema. The cystostomy tube is closed 24 h after surgery and removed when the child passes urine spontaneously. The dressing is removed 24–48 h after surgery. All steps of the procedure are depicted in Fig. 8.3a and b.

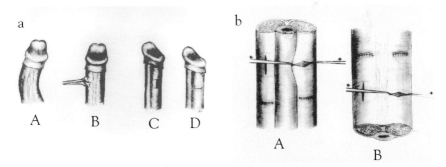

Figure 8.3. (a) Steps in the technique of incisional corporoplasty: A, artificial erection after degloving of the penile skin, showing the lateral curvature; B, preview of the straightening of the curvature by applying Allis clamps to the most convex part of the tunica albuginea; C, longitudinal incision of the tunica using a no. 11 scalpel blade held with its cutting edge upwards to prevent injury to the cavernous tissues; D, horizontal suturing of the longitudinal incision in order to shorten the convex part of the tunica. (b) Position of the incisions in dorsal and ventral curvatures: A, straightening of dorsal curvature by horizontal closure of the longitudinal incisions made at both sides of the corpus spongiosum; B, straightening of ventral curvature by horizontal closure of the longitudinal incisions made at both sides of the neurovascular bundle.

Results

Nineteen children with congenital penile curvature were treated by this technique, all successfully (Fig. 8.4). This corporoplasty technique was also used in 14 cases of hypospadias to straighten residual curvature after complete excision of chordee.

Discussion

As no tissue segments have to be removed from the tunica albuginea, there is no risk of injuring or scarring the erectile tissues. In the classic Nesbit procedure[4] and the Nesbit-Kelami modification,[5] segments of the tunica have to be excised and dissected from the underlying erectile tissues, increasing the risk of scarring these tissues. For the same reason, in the technique described here, the scarring of the tunica at the site of the incisions is minimal, preventing curvature towards the repaired side during the development of the penis. In five of the children who were 8–9 years old at the time of the repair, after 2 to 3 years follow-up no such curvature was observed.

Use of this technique obviates the need to mobilize the neurovascular bundle and the corpus spongiosum to remove segments from the tunica albuginea. As the incisions in the tunica are parallel to these structures, the risk of injuring them is minimal. In the author's opinion, penile curvature in children, like hypospadias, should be treated at as early a stage as possible in order to prevent the psychosexual consequences of this abnormality.

a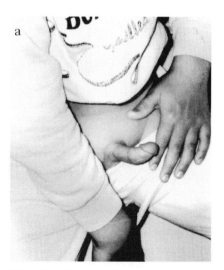

b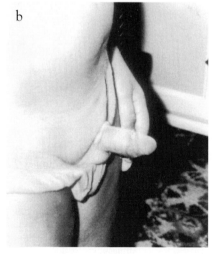

Figure 8.4. (a) Dorsal penile curvature in an 8-year-old patient; (b) complete straightening of the penis, as seen 45 days after incisional corporoplasty.

References

1. Yachia D, Beyar M, Aridogan I A, Descalu S. Incidence of penile curvatures. J Urol 1993; 150: 1478–1479
2. Yachia D. Modified corporoplasty for the treatment of penile curvature. J Urol 1990; 143: 80–82
3. Yachia D. Early assessment of penile curvatures in infants. J Urol 1991; 145: 103–104
4. Nesbit R M. Congenital curvature of the phallus: report of three cases with description of corrective operation. J Urol 1965; 93: 230–232
5. Kelami A. Congenital penile deviation and its treatment with Nesbit-Kelami technique. Br J Urol 1987; 60: 261–263

9

Micropenis: evaluation and approach

N. G. Prado   E. Ide   A. J. Batista

Introduction

During the last decade there have been many reports of micropenis, which is a long-standing problem, involving different concepts and various types of morphology, such as micropenis, microphallus, palmate, buried or concealed penis, webbed penis and penoscrotal fusion, transposition or malposition (Fig. 9.1). The term micropenis is used for those organs that fall more than 2.5 standard deviations below the norm for the age.[1,3] In brief, micropenis is defined as a stretched penis length (see later) less than 2.0 cm at birth, 2.5 cm at one year, 4.0 cm in the prepubertal adolescent and 10 cm in the postpubertal adolescent or adult.

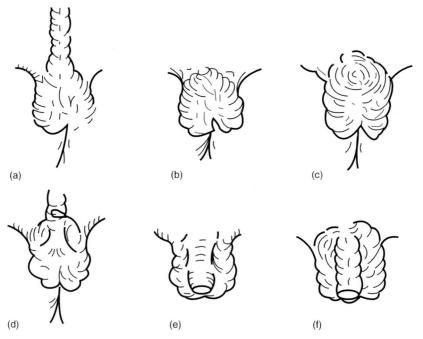

(a)

(b)

(c)

(d)

(e)

(f)

Figure 9.1. Penoscrotal malformation: (a) normal; (b) palmate penis; (c) buried/concealed penis; (d) high scrotal implantation; (e) webbed penis; (f) penoscrotal transposition or fusion.

During the first trimester of gestation under the influence of foetal Leydig activity (androgenic), differentiation of the phallus with male characteristics is complete, but continues. After week 14 of gestation the penis grows tenfold under androgenic stimulation, failure of which results in a perfectly formed but small penis.[2] Tables 9.1 and 9.2 list the causes of micropenis and comparative findings in anomalous, endocrinous and intersexual microphallus.[1,2]

Cause	Type
Endocrine	Primary testicular
	End organ
	Hypothalamic–pituitary
	Pituitary growth hormone
	? Acquired suppression
Non-endocrine	Defective morphogenesis

Data from reference 2.

Table 9.1. Causes of microphallus (micropenis)

	Anomalous	Hypogonadotrophic	Hypospadias
Prepuce			
Normal		X	
Thickened	X		
Dorsal			X
Glans			
Proportional		X	X
Small	X		
Meatus			
Normal		X	
Within prepuce	X		
Ventral			X
Internal genitalia			
Normal	X		
Immature		X	
Feminized			X

Data from reference 2.

Table 9.2. Comparative findings in anomalous, endocrine and intersexual micropenis

At birth the penis has attained 26% of the mean adult penile length. The mean diameter of the penis at birth is 1.1 cm.[3] Table 9.3 gives the mean (stretched) penile length of normal male subjects of various ages.

The principal task when investigating children with micropenis is to determine whether it is a true micropenis due to systemic endocrinopathy, androgen insensitivity (receptor blocking), or a familial and obstetric disorder (hypospadias, cryptorchidism, Kollman's or Prader-Willi syndrome), or else a normal-sized penis that is anatomically malformed or malpositioned. To confirm the diagnosis of micropenis the paediatrician or urologist must have a reference point; it is very important to differentiate between true micropenis and a penis that is normally formed but small in size. The size of the penis is determined by measuring the stretched length with a rigid ruler. A small ruler is placed on the pubic ramus, with a depressed fat pad, and the glans penis is grasped firmly and stretched. The length of the penis is read along the dorsum from the pubis to the tip of the glans. During this procedure, palpation to assess development of the corpora and measurement of the mid-shaft diameter should be included in the examination.[4] The length of the penis measured in this way has been found to correlate closely with the length of the penis in the erect state.

Age	Penile length (cm)	
	Mean ±SD	Mean −2.5 SD
Newborn (30 weeks)	2.5 ± 0.4*	1.5*
Newborn (34 weeks)	3.0 ± 0.4*	2.0*
0–5 months	3.9 ± 0.8	1.9
6–12 months	4.3 ± 0.8	2.3
1–2 years	4.7 ± 0.8	2.6
2–3 years	5.1 ± 0.9	2.9
3–4 years	5.5 ± 0.9	3.3
4–5 years	5.7 ± 0.9	3.5
5–6 years	6.0 ± 0.9	3.8
6–7 years	6.1 ± 0.9	3.9
7–8 years	6.2 ± 1.0	3.7
8–9 years	6.3 ± 1.0	3.8
9–10 years	6.3 ± 1.0	3.8
10–11 years	6.4 ± 1.1	3.7
Adult	13.3 ± 1.6	9.3

*From Feldman and Smith. Remainder from Schonfed and Beebe

Table 9.3. Stretched penile length in normal male subjects

In a rare situation, a karyotype study should be performed in a child; however, gonadotrophin studies must be conducted routinely to determine the functional integrity of the hypothalamic–pituitary-testicular axis.[5,6]

Patients and technique

From January 1986 to March 1994, 12 boys, aged 3 to 10 years, presenting with micropenis because of the mal-positioned penile, underwent surgical correction. Indications for surgery varied from unsatisfactory appearance of the penis to almost complete penoscrotal transposition.

Surgical repair of a penis that appears small because of anomalous penoscrotal pubic insertion has not been well defined, although there are some reports of penoscrotal transposition.[7–13] The authors' surgical procedure to correct mild to all but the most severe types of malpositioned penis are based on the same surgical principle, outlined below.

The penis is inspected carefully. In most cases, the corporal and urethral bodies, as well as the glans, are normal: the defect is related only to a different penile site, the penile pubic insertion being below the scrotal implantation (Fig. 9.2a). The malpositioned penis, which appears to be small, is hidden by the bulk of the scrotum and subsequently by inadequate anchorage of the penile skin to the deep fascia. The penis is repositioned through a vertical and transverse (H-shaped) suprapubic incision by removing skin and fat (in obese patients) from the dorsal base of the penis to the pubic symphysis and by creation of asymmetrical lateral flaps with relocation of the scrotal compartment in a normal position (Fig. 9.2b, c). Elastic tissue is incised, any fat is excised en bloc, and the symphysis is cleared of areolar tissue. Absorbable sutures are placed through the skin and subcutaneous tissue at the upper site to form the base of the penis and are anchored to the deep fascia or in some cases to the periosteum of the pubis. If phimosis is present, a coronal circumcizing incision is made and the surgical procedure is performed. On the ventral shaft of the penis, all fibrous tissue is excised if necessary and the lateral scrotal flaps are brought together beneath the phallus (Fig. 9.2d, e). The incision is closed in one layer with 4/0 absorbable interrupted sutures. A compression dressing impregnated with antibiotic ointment is applied for 48–72 h. General anaesthesia is administered; a Foley catheter was inserted in only one patient.

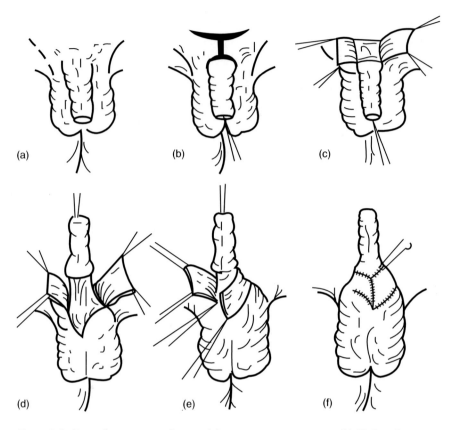

Figure 9.2. Surgical correction technique: (a) preoperative appearance; (b) H-shaped incision; (c) releasing the dorsal base of the penis; (d) creation of asymmetrical flaps; (e) lateral flaps moved down to the ventral shaft of the penis; (f) final cosmetic appearance.

Discussion

The term 'micropenis' has been widely used to refer to a small penile appearance independent of its aetiology. True micropenis may be classified as occurring both in those with endocrinological failure and those without endocrinopathy (idiopathic). In both groups of patients, the glans penis, although diminutive, is normal and the urethra and meatus are normally positioned.[3,4] The traditional treatment for true micropenis has been hormone therapy (human chorionic gonadotrophin, testosterone) but a surgical repair technique has been reported recently.[13,14]

Surgical treatment is appropriate when a newborn or infant boy is diagnosed as having a small penis. The parents' first concern is undoubtedly the cosmetic appearance of the genitalia. The appearance affects the parental attitude and this, in turn, influences the child's self-perception. In most cases, the parents are firm in their desire to have the condition corrected surgically.

All 12 children treated by the authors had a pleasing cosmetic appearance postoperatively; there was no instance of skin problem, infection, dehiscence or any other complication. Urinary diversion by urethral catheter was necessary in one patient only.

Even in the case of only a slightly malpositioned penis, surgery by the techniques described above is indicated by the abnormal appearance of the penis and the wishes of the parents. In the authors' opinion, elective penile surgery should be performed at as early a stage as possible, for cosmetic and psychological reasons. Their new approach, for correction of a small penis caused by abnormal penoscrotal insertion, results in a penis of adequate appearance and satisfactory length.

As the normal condition is more thoroughly investigated and becomes better understood and defined, so a greater number of abnormalities may be diagnosed at birth or soon after. During this period, aesthetic correction of structural genital abnormalities is probably the greatest concern for the physician, the parents and the patients.

References

1. Aaronson I A. Micropenis: medical and surgical implications. J Urol 1994; 152: 4–14
2. Hinman F Jr. Microphallus: distinction between anomalous and endocrine types. J Urol 1980; 123: 412–415
3. Diagnosis and therapy of micropenis. Micropenis. Dialogues in Pediatric Urology 1984; 7: No. 1
4. Lee P A, Mazur T, Danish R, Amrhein J, Blizzard R M, Money J, Migeon C J. Micropenis. I. Criteria, etiologies and classification. John Hopkins Med J 1980; 146: 156–163
5. Kogan S J, Williams D I. The micropenis syndrome: clinical observations and expectations for growth. J Urol 1977; 118: 311–313
6. Penile growth. Micropenis and penile growth: understanding the underlying factors. Dialogues in Pediatric Urology 1994; 17: No. 5
7. Glenn J F, Anderson E E. Surgical correction of incomplete penoscotal transposition. J Urol 1973; 110: 603–605
8. Maizels M, Zaontz M, Donovan J, Bushnick P N, Firlit C F. Surgical correction of the buried penis: description of a classification system and a techique to correct the disorder. J Urol 1986; 136: 268–271
9. Webbed penis. J Urol 1974; 111: 690–692
10. Redman J F. A technique for the correction of penoscrotal fusion. J Urol 1985; 133: 432–433
11. Shapiro S R. Surgical treatment of the 'buried' penis. Urology 1987; 30: 554–559
12. Shiraki I W, Shirai R S. Congenital micropenile skin sleeve. J Urol 1975; 114: 469–472

13. Burkholder G V, Newell M E. New surgical treatment for micropenis. J Urol 1980; 129: 832–834
14. Jones H W Jr, Park I J, Rock J A. Technique for surgical sex reassignment for micropenis and allied conditions. Am J Obstet Gynecol 1978; 132: 870–877

REPORT

Penile reconstruction in exstrophy and epispadias

10

C.R.J. Woodhouse

Introduction

Epispadias, classical exstrophy and its variations, and cloacal exstrophy form a spectrum of malformations in the development of the cloaca and genitalia. In the male, malformation of the penis is an integral part of the complex: it has an open, epispadiac urethra; its corpora are short; the attachments to the inferior pubic ramus are abnormal, and there is tight dorsal chordee on erection. Although the severity of the abnormalities varies from one end of the exstrophy spectrum to the other, the basic anatomy is the same in all cases of exstrophy and epispadias with an open pelvic ring. Successful reconstruction depends on an understanding of these anatomical details.

Genital anatomy

The orientation of the inferior pubic rami and the attachments of the deep parts of the corpora are unlike those of normal males. The findings by cavernosogram, by computerized tomography (CT) and surgical exploration are consistent.[1] Not only is the symphysis open but the pelvis is rotated caudally, so that the inferior pubic ramus is parallel to the floor when the patient is standing (Fig. 10.1).

The oblique view of the pelvis gives a true lateral view of the inferior pubic ramus. The orientation of the inferior pubic rami is seen in Fig. 10.2. A cavernosogram in this projection shows that the deep parts of the corpora are, similarly, lying horizontally.

Comparison of the cavernosograms and CT scans in exstrophy with those of normal men shows the reason for the shortness of the penis; it is not, as might be thought, that the symphysis is open causing most of the penis to be buried in the perineum; the corpora are actually deficient in length, although of normal calibre.

Further evidence for this view has been provided by the results of surgical apposition of the pubic bones in infancy. In cases reported by Johnston[2] and in the author's own cases, those who had successful

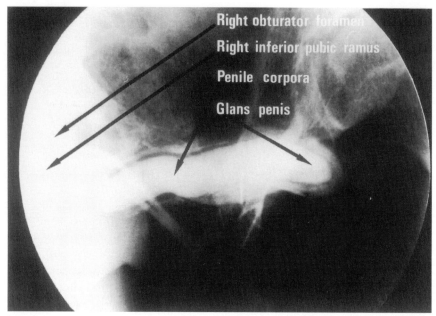

Right obturator foramen
Right inferior pubic ramus
Penile corpora
Glans penis

Figure 10.1. Oblique view of a cavernosogram in an exstrophy patient showing the relationship of the corpora to the pubis. Note that the penis is parallel to the floor. (Reproduced from ref. 26 with permission.)

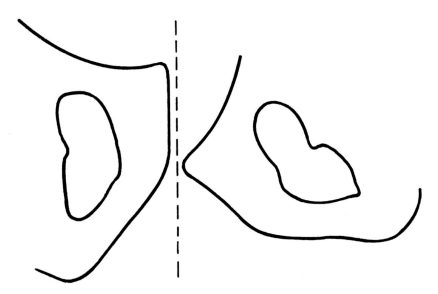

Figure 10.2. Diagram of the pelvic orientation: left, normal and right, exstrophy. (Reproduced from ref. 26 with permission.)

apposition of the pubis as part of their original bladder closure do not have a longer penis than others. However, it has been pointed out that the penis is longer if the divarication of the pubic bones is 3 cm or less and it is shorter if the divarication is 4 cm or more.[3]

McLorie et al.[4] have tried to establish an experimental model for the penile deformity using an inflatable penile prosthesis attached to a normal adult pelvis. They demonstrated that the visible penis was longer when the pubic ring was closed. It seems unlikely that these findings can be translated to the abnormal penis and pelvis of exstrophy.

The blood supply of the exstrophic penis has not been fully investigated, but the flow of contrast into the veins that occurs with cavernosography, and the operative findings, suggest that the blood supply of such a penis is normal. The main supply (and certainly the main venous drainage) appears to come from the pudendal vessels passing through Alcock's canal. There is no cross-circulation between the corpora.

Dissection of an infant with cloacal exstrophy who died 72 days after birth has produced some interesting information. The arterial supply to the penis was from pudendal arteries that travelled in the perineum, with the somatic nerves, to supply the corpora. The venous drainage travelled subcutaneously through the inguinal canals and into the external iliacs. The autonomic nerves lay in the midline in front of the sacrum and then split to pierce the pelvic floor on each side, medial and posterior to the bladder.[5] Obviously, it is uncertain how much of this anatomy is applicable to the classical exstrophy.

The position of the superficial neurovascular bundles reflects the lateral rotation or 'kippering' of the corpora. They lie in the true lateral position in the distal and middle portions of the corpora, moving dorso-laterally as they pass proximally (Fig. 10.3).[6]

The urethral plate is on the dorsum of the penis and is, by definition, open. Surgical dissection in adults suggests that there is a layer of erectile tissue running along the proximal two-thirds of the ventral aspect, corresponding to the corpus spongiosum.

The fate of the bulbospongiosus muscle is unknown. Logic would suggest that it is present in some form. It might well be too small to identify in the neonate and perhaps destroyed in the primary reconstruction. The author has not seen any sign of it in adults.

The prostate is present. In the initial dissection in the neonate it is detached from the penile urethra and remains in its normal relationship to the bladder base. In a series of 13 adult men (four of whom were continent) assessed by magnetic resonance imaging, the prostate was found to have a mean weight of 21.7 g, which is normal for age. In all

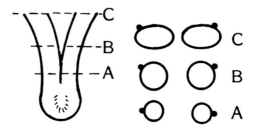

Figure 10.3. Diagrams of the anatomy of the superficial neurovascular bundles in exstrophy: (left) dorsal view of the penis; (right) transverse sections at the levels indicated showing the bundles. (Reproduced from ref. 26 with permission.)

cases the prostate was posterior to the urethra so that it could not provide any outflow resistance. The puborectalis muscles were widely separated.[7] The verumontanum, which is normally positioned, is a useful landmark for surgery in later life.

Appearances in adults

The adult epispadiac penis is short (Fig. 10.4). It often appears broad because of the separation of the corpora but is, in fact, of normal calibre. The abnormalities may be exaggerated by the recession of the suprapubic area, absence of the mons pubis and normal size of the scrotum.

At birth, the pubic hairbearing skin is displaced laterally. Modern reconstruction attempts a midline closure so that the hair grows as a normal triangular escutcheon, but this is not always successful. In the older reconstructions with W-shaped skin flaps and in newer types of

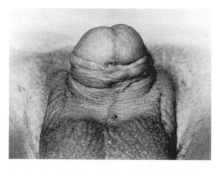
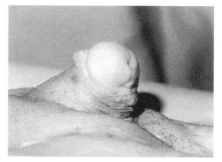

Figure 10.4. Clinical photographs of the adult flaccid exstrophy penis; left: ventral view, right: lateral view.

closure with a less than perfect result, the pubic hair lies on either side of the pubic area (Fig. 10.5).

The shape of the erect penis depends on the initial reconstruction. In the natural state, the erect epispadiac penis has a tight dorsal chordee (Fig. 10.6). A cavernosogram in these cases shows that the site of the maximum curvature is at the point where the corpora emerge from the perineum.[8] Increasing awareness of this problem has modified the reconstruction in infancy[9] to produce a more normal angle of erection.

The degree of chordee is variable. In some the angle is such that sexual intercourse is possible either in the conventional position or in one that brings the female introitus into more direct apposition to the penis.

It might be thought that this deformity was due to the scar tissue around the dorsally placed urethra. It has been said that clearance of the scar and detachment of the urethra corrects the chordee,[10] but the author has found this to be so in only one of 32 patients coming to operation. Although the original problem may have been a congenitally short urethral plate, by adulthood the basic problem is intrinsic curvature of the corpora. The penile dissections in infancy and childhood may modify the erectile deformity, for better or for worse.

A more complex deformity occurs when one or both of the corpora are damaged in the initial surgery so that they fail to fill completely. If one corpus fails to fill on erection it acts on the other as a 'bowstring' and causes lateral deviation, in addition to the dorsal chordee.[8]

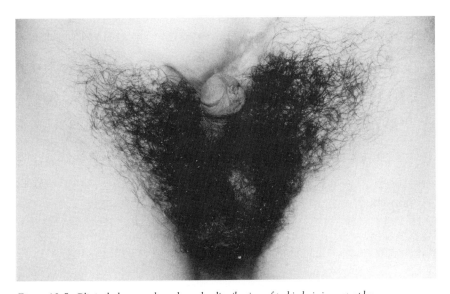

Figure 10.5. Clinical photograph to show the distribution of pubic hair in exstrophy.

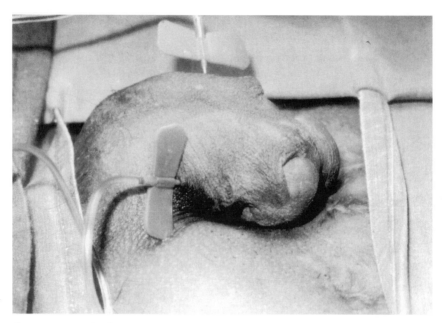

Figure 10.6. Artificial erection to show tight dorsal chordee in an extrophy penis.

If both corpora are rudimentary, the visible or exophytic part of the penis is normal, except that it is a little higher than usual on the abdomen. On cavernosography the corpora appear to have no attachment to the pubic rami; erection is very limited and the penis unstable. In one of the author's patients the whole of one corpus and the exophytic part of the other is missing, so that there is no visible penis at all.

The evidence suggests that the corpora are normal at birth and are damaged at the primary (and revision) reconstructive surgery.[1,11] The distribution of types of erectile deformity currently seen in adult exstrophy patients is shown in Table 10.1.

Awareness of the erectile problems and appropriate reconstruction in infancy may improve the function in adults. Although the techniques

Abnormality	Incidence (%)
Dorsal chordee	77
Unilateral rudimentary corpus	9
Bilateral rudimentary corpus	14

Table 10.1. Incidence of erectile deformities in exstrophy and epispadias

reviewed by Snyder[9] have not been in use for long enough to allow adult follow-up, results from the Mayo Clinic suggest that modern techniques of reconstruction do lead to just this situation: a short but normal penis with a normal angle of erection was found in 24 of 44 adults.[12]

Investigation

An artificial erection, either by intracorporeal injections of papaverine or by infusion, will demonstrate the erectile deformity, but it will not define the anatomy of the deep portion of the corpora. Unless the patient describes an uncomplicated dorsal chordee and the deep parts of the corpora are palpably normal, a cavernosogram is essential.

The cavernosogram technique is modified from that described by Herzberg et al.[13] The corpora must be infused separately because of the absence of cross-circulation; 120 ml 65% urograffin in 250 ml physiological saline is used. A pressure of 300 mmHg is generated by Fenwall bags. The corpora are punctured with 19 gauge butterfly needles. No tourniquet should be used as it would obscure the true chordee that occurs in the deep part of the corpora.[8]

Lengthening procedures

The anatomical evidence, outlined above, shows that the corpora are deficient in length. Increase in the length of the visible penis can be achieved only by making the best use of the corpora distal to their attachment to the inferior pubic ramus. Some additional length may be achieved by osteotomy to close the pubic symphysis in the first few days of life. Whatever the situation in infants, pelvic osteotomy does not seem to be a very attractive option for adults. As previously mentioned, those who had an osteotomy in infancy as a part of their primary repair have not retained the apposition into adolescence and do not have a longer penis than others.[2]

In some patients the corpora may have been concertinaed by contraction and scarring of the urethral plate and pericorporeal tissue. Considerable lengthening can be achieved in children by clearing all this tissue away and cleaning the corpora.[14] This dissection is the first step in chordee correction but in the author's experience in adults it has not allowed any penile lengthening; it may be that, by this stage in life, secondary and irreversible changes have occurred in the corpora.

The horizontal plane in which the inferior pubic rami lie prevents the lengthening of the penis by partial detachment of the corpora. Some length is gained by dissection from the body of the pubis but it is useless to continue it posterior to the junction with the inferior ramus.

Complete detachment of the corpora from the inferior pubic rami is said to have given good lengthening in nine of 11 children.[15,16] However, there has been no follow-up and the procedure could damage the blood supply reaching the corpora through Alcock's canal.

Thus, it seems that in adolescents and adults there is no worthwhile procedure to lengthen the penis. Good chordee correction will give a little increase in length and will allow the best use to be made of the length that is available.

Appreciation of the erectile deformities has stimulated better reconstruction in infants. Maximum possible release of the corpora and correction of the chordee by the Cantwell–Ransley technique (see below) can produce a near-normal penis in childhood. Perovic et al.[17] have reported that the penis in infants is similar in length to that of normal boys, although slightly different in appearance.

Correction of erectile deformities

Selection

Ideally, the penile anomaly should be corrected at the time of the initial reconstruction in infancy. Release of the urethral plate and chordee and partial detachment of the corpora from the pubis are considered essential steps.[9] It is rare for correction to be completed in a single stage, the mean being 1.62 operations (range 1–4).[12] It is best to achieve complete reconstruction in infancy and to allow the child to grow up looking as much like his peers as possible. The appearance and function of the penis are of paramount importance to the adolescent with exstrophy.[18] There must be a word of caution, however. The complex erectile deformities that the author has seen in some patients are due to rudimentary corpora; it is most likely that they were normal at birth and were damaged by surgery in infancy. Although there are now many techniques to reconstruct a near-normal bladder de novo, so far there is no operation to restore the corpora, let alone construct a penis with sexual sensation and function.

The patients who are now adults have some degree of erectile deformity and many require phalloplasty. Careful selection is important. It is preferable to wait until penile growth is complete at the end of puberty and also until the boy has developed emotionally so that he understands the purpose of the operation. It is not satisfactory to embark on a programme of cosmetic operations if the patient cannot see anything wrong with the existing situation. If he has an understanding partner and has tried to have intercourse, it is a help, but in the author's opinion it is unwise to wait until repeated failures have damaged the patient's ego.

Reconstruction

Several methods of correcting the deformities of the exstrophic penis have been described. If the deformity is considered as a curve in a parallel-sided cylinder, two basic methods are available for its correction: lengthening the concave side or shortening the convex side. The techniques developed for Peyronie's disease are applicable.

Shortening of the convexity is relatively simple by Nesbit's procedure. No dissection on the dorsum is required. The urethra normally lies on the dorsum and so will not be affected by the surgery.

Lengthening of the concavity by implantation of some material in the corpora produces slight lengthening (Fig. 10.7). In Peyronie's disease many autologous and heterologous materials have been used; in exstrophy only the use of skin and of lyophilized dura mater have been reported. The results of using dura have been good and it is therefore disappointing to find that sterilization may not kill all the viruses in the material. A case has been reported of Jakob–Creutzfeld disease developing in a 28-year-old woman who had received a dural graft 22 months earlier.[19] Although different processes are followed by manufacturers, all preparations may carry a risk of transmitting this viral disease. If one virus can be carried, presumably others can also. When an implant is needed, skin, rectus sheath or tunica vaginalis may be used instead of dura.[11,20,21]

The Koff procedure is an ingenious method of rotating the corpora so that their curvatures cancel out and the resulting angle of erection is satisfactory.[22] The technique has been modified and is commonly known as the Cantwell–Ransley operation (Fig. 10.8). Reports in infants and adolescents show that the short-term results are very good and the complication rate low. Gearhart et al.[23] have used this technique in 26 infants, all of whom have had a good cosmetic result.

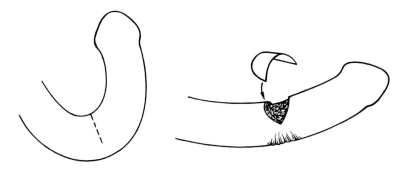

Figure 10.7. Diagram to show the principle of tissue inlay in the dorsum of the penis to correct chordee. (Reproduced from ref. 26 with permission.)

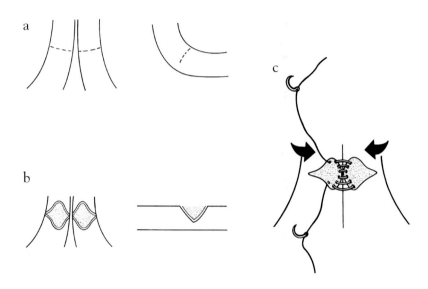

Figure 10.8. The Cantwell–Ransley operation: steps in a rotational phalloplasty: (a) the incision in the corpora seen from the dorsum and laterally; (b) the corpora straightened out; (c) the corpora rotated towards each other and the openings in the corpora sutured together face to face. (Reproduced from ref. 26 with permission.)

The indications for the various reconstructions are shown in Table 10.2.

The urethra

The urethral plate in exstrophy is on the dorsum of the penis and is too short. Current techniques of reconstruction allow for division of the plate and urethroplasty. Modern reconstruction in infants transfers the

Abnormality	Technique advocated
Dorsal chordee	
Mild	Nesbit's
Major (minimal separation)	Cantwell–Ransley
Major (wide separation)	Inlay rectus sheath
Single rudimentary corpus	Inlay rectus sheath + Nesbit's
Bilateral rudimentary corpus	Leave alone

Table 10.2. Current concepts for correction of erectile deformity in epispadias

urethra to the ventrum. This gives a more natural appearance and contributes to the correction of chordee.[23]

In an adult the urethra is nearly always too short for phalloplasty; the author uses the length available to form a urethrostomy at the penoscrotal junction. Urethroplasty is performed at a second stage, if the patient wishes, by rolling a tube out of ventral skin to bring the meatus to the tip of the glans. In the author's experience, the complication rate is high: even when the short-term result is good, it is difficult to keep a 'dry' urethra patent; patients frequently develop strictures resulting in absent ejaculation and sometimes in painful orgasm.

There is seldom enough skin to allow urethroplasty at the same time as penile straightening. On two occasions in patients with urinary diversion there has been enough bladder remaining to mobilize a strip of urothelium and detrusor on a pedicle from the bladder neck area. The strip is rolled into a tube and brought to the tip of the glans as a urethra.[24]

Of 13 urethroplasties in diverted patients, only six have achieved a complete urethra without any fistula or stricture. The remainder have been left with at least one small fistula (or worse) and have declined further reconstruction. Such poor results do not encourage patients to undergo secondary urethroplasty.

The mons pubis

In adult exstrophy patients at present, the pubic area is nearly always recessed from the uncorrected divarication of the pubic bones. The pubic hair lies on either side of the midline.

It is most important, either in infancy or in adolescence, to rotate hairbearing flaps of skin and fat to cover the midline defect. The flaps may be based laterally or inferiorly (Fig. 10.9).[25,26] Although the inferiorly based flaps have been described for females only, they should be equally applicable to males. If too little skin is available, larger flaps can be created by the use of skin expanders.[27]

Sexual function

With or without surgical correction, men appear to have a normal libido. If the penis is straight enough, most are able to have penetrative sexual intercourse. Mesrobian et al.[12] report 83% of men having satisfactory intercourse with reconstruction only in infancy.[12] They have fewer casual sexual partners than would be expected; they appear to form very stable partnerships with normal women and have a normal family life.

Although complete reconstruction in infancy is desirable, later surgery also produces a satisfactory sexual outcome. Using a variety of

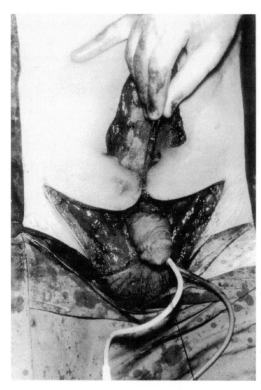

Figure 10.9. Operative photograph to show the laterally based, pubic hairbearing skin flaps being rotated to the mons veneris. (The patient has also had a midline hernia repaired with plastic mesh, which can be seen in the wound. He also has two urethrae, which have been catheterized.)

techniques, Audry *et al.*[28] established normal function in seven of 14 adolescents or adults. With the Cantwell–Ransley technique, four of seven adolescents are able to achieve normal intercourse.[17] Obviously, those who were not having intercourse in these series may yet establish sexual relationships.

Of 43 patients in the author's series for whom full information is available, 33 have been married or lived with a partner, although most required some reconstruction in adolescence. Only one patient is known to be homosexual and he is one of three who have gone into the priesthood. One boy has doubts about his sexual identity and he is an epispadiac rather than a true case of exstrophy; he may come to gender reassignment eventually. The remaining patients of all ages do not admit to any sexual contact and for many of them the combination of abnormal genitalia and an external urinary diversion seems to be too overwhelming.[29]

The effect of changing an ileal conduit for an internal continent diversion is striking. The author is aware of young men who lived a celibate existence, apparently because of their abnormal penis. Internal continent diversion subsequently gave them sufficient self-confidence to develop relationships with women. For the next generation a working bladder and counselling of children and parents may further improve sexual function.

A case has been made for early gender reassignment for male infants with grossly deficient penis and exstrophy, especially cloacal exstrophy. In the view of King,[30] this might cover 20% of cases. Cases have been cited where refusal of such advice by the parents has resulted in poorly adjusted adolescents who commit sexual offences (McLorie et al. 1991).[4] In a series of eight males with cloacal exstrophy, only one achieved successful vaginal intercourse; two were impotent and three required intensive psychiatric counselling.[31] One of the author's patients, whose penis is reasonably sized for exstrophy, has served a prison sentence for attempted rape.

Young boys with exstrophy can certainly be converted into girls very successfully.[30] However, there has been no long-term follow-up of exstrophy patients reassigned to the female gender and it is possible that they will make equally unhappy female adolescents. In the author's experience, with appropriate help, males with a very small penis attributable to any cause can have a satisfactory life as a male. Sexual intercourse and other relations with female partners have been normal. The author's series includes an exstrophy patient whose penis was gradually destroyed in reconstructive operations in another hospital: he is left with only the deep part of the left corpus and no visible penis. He is well adjusted and, aged 23, started a stable sexual relationship with a girl; they appear to have a mutually satisfactory sex life.

The author is not of the opinion that male infants should be turned into girls just because the penis is small.

Ejaculation

Ejaculation has been assessed continuously during follow-up. In the first review of adult patients, all but two of 31 patients ejaculated.[31] Absence of ejaculation is still rare, in spite of the more extensive reconstructions that are done, but the emission that does occur is slow and may continue over several hours after orgasm.

In another series, 16 of 25 patients had ejaculation but its quality is not recorded.[12] Some patients with a diversion and a dry bladder describe a more-or-less continuous urethral discharge of semen-like fluid. Analysis suggests that this is a mixture of semen, pus and prostatic secretion.

Although the genital tract up to the verumontanum is normal, there is a high incidence of poor or absent sperm. It is not known whether this is due to obstruction or repeated infection. The data in Table 10.3 show that patients who had an early diversion have better sperm than those in whom reconstruction was attempted.

Semen quality	Exstrophy		Epispadias	
	Reconst**	Diversion	Reconst	Diversion
No ejaculation	1			
Azoospermia	9	16		
Poor	5	6	4[†]	
Good	2	11	3	6
Paternity[‡]	1	5		

*Data from refs 29, 31 and 33.
**Reconst = reconstructed bladder.
[†]Diversion or reconstruction not stated.
[‡]Men who claim to have fathered children have not had semen analyses.

Table 10.3. Seminal analysis of patients with exstrophy or epispadias*

Paternity

In a review of adult exstrophy patients, the author reported that seven of 44 patients had initiated one or two pregnancies from which there have been five children; a further 13 were known to be infertile.[26] These figures were broadly in line with those reported elsewhere: Mesrobian et al.[12] report 12 of 53 patients married, five of whom had fathered children. In a later generation of patients from this institution, the figures have changed little.[32]

The main cause of infertility appears to be repeated prostatic and bladder infections. Thus, ironically, the boys who underwent early urinary diversion have the best record for fertility.[33]

It has been reported from a postal survey of clinics throughout the world, that one in 70 offspring of exstrophy or epispadias patients, themselves have the condition.[34] This figure must represent the worst that can be expected. In the large series describing the obstetric record of exstrophic females and in those describing male sexual function, there is no record of any offspring having exstrophy or epispadias. These papers, together with the author's own patients, include 81 normal babies.[12,35,37]

Sexually transmitted diseases

Although exstrophy patients tend to grow up with a strong sense of social and family responsibility,[29] they are not immune from the complications of sexual activity. In the patients attending the author's clinic, three examples of the latter have been seen. One young man managed to fracture his corpus during vigorous penetration. It failed to heal spontaneously after 4 weeks and, after localized surgical repair, he was impotent for several months, but eventually returned to normal. In the author's experience, this has been the only case of cross-circulation between the corpora; it probably resulted from the trauma. The author has also seen one case of gonococcal pyocystis, in a patient with an ileal conduit diversion. In addition, one young man contracted extensive venereal warts (Fig. 10.10)

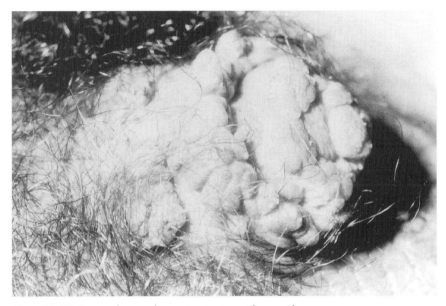

Figure 10.10. A case of venereal warts in a patient with exstrophy.

References

1. Woodhouse C R J, Kellett M J. Anatomy of the penis and its deformities in exstrophy and epispadias. J Urol 1984; 132: 1122–1124

2. Johnston J H. Lengthening of the congenital or acquired short penis. Br J Urol 1974; 46: 685–687

3. Schillinger J F, Wiley M J. Bladder exstrophy penile lengthening procedure. Urology 1984; 24: 434–437

4. McLorie G A, Bellemore M C, Salter R B. Penile deformity in bladder exstrophy: correlation with closure of the pelvic defect. J Pediatr Surg 1991; 26: 201–203

5. Schlegel P N, Gearhart J P. Neuroanatomy of the pelvis in an infant with cloacal exstrophy: a detailed microdissection with histology. J Urol 1989; 141: 583–585

6. Hurwitz R S, Woodhouse C R J, Ransley P G. The anatomical course of the neurovascular bundles in epispadias. J Urol 1986; 136: 68–70

7. Gearhart J P, Young A, Leonard M P et al. Prostate size and configuration in adults with bladder exstrophy. J Urol 1993; 149: 308–310

8. Woodhouse C R J. The management of erectile deformity in adults with exstrophy and epispadias. J Urol 1986; 135: 932–935

9. Snyder H M. Epispadias and exstrophy. In: Whitfield H N (ed) Rob and Smith's Operative surgery — genito urinary surgery. Oxford: Butterworth-Heinemann, 1993: 786–813

10. Spehr C, Melchior C. Operative correction of the penis deformity in bladder exstrophy. XXth Congress of the International Society of Urology, Vienna, 1985: 320 (abstr 1008)

11. Brzezinski A E, Homsy Y L, Laberge I. Orthoplasty in epispadias. J Urol 1986; 136: 259–261

12. Mesrobian H-G J, Kelalis P P, Kramer S A. Long term follow-up of cosmetic appearance and genital function in boys with exstrophy: review of 53 patients. J Urol 1986; 136: 256–258

13. Herzberg Z, Kellett M J, Morgan R J, Pryor J P. Method, indications and results of corpus cavernosography. Br J Urol 1981; 53: 641–644

14. Hendren W H. Penile lengthening after previous repair of epispadias. J Urol 1979; 121: 527–534

15. Kelley J H, Eraklis A J. A procedure for lengthening the phallus in boys with exstrophy of the bladder. J Pediatr Surg 1971; 6: 645–649

16. King L R. Editorial: exstrophy and epispadias. J Urol 1984; 132: 1159–1160

17. Perovic S, Scepanovic D, Sremcevic D, Vukadinovic V. Epispadias surgery — Belgrade experience. Br J Urol 1992; 70: 674–677

18. Feinberg T, Lattimer J K, Jeter K et al. Questions that worry children with exstrophy. Pediatrics 1974; 53: 242–246

19. Editorial. Update: Creutzfeld–Jacob disease in a patient receiving a cadaveric dura mater graft. JAMA 1987; 258: 309–310

20. Bruschini H, Mitre A I. Peyronie's disease: surgical treatment with muscular aponeurosis. Urology 1979; 13: 505–508

21. Das S. Peyronie's disease: excision and autografting with tunica vaginalis. J Urol 1980; 124: 818–821

22. Koff S A, Eakins M. The treatment of penile chordee using corporeal rotation. J Urol 1984; 131: 931–932

23. Gearhart J P, Leonard M P, Burgers J K, Jeffs R D. The Cantwell–Ransley technique for repair of epispadias. J Urol 1992; 148: 851–854

24. Woodhouse C R J. Dural phalloplasty in exstrophy and epispadias. In: Mundy A R (ed) Current operative surgery — urology. London: Ballière Tindall, 1988: 106–118

25. Ship A G, Pelzer R H. Reconstruction of the female escutcheon in exstrophy of the bladder. Plast Reconstr Surg 1972; 49: 643–646

26. Woodhouse C R J. Long-term paediatric urology. Oxford: Blackwell Scientific Publications, 1991: 127–150

27. Marconi F, Messina P, Pavanello P, DeCastro R. Cosmetic reconstruction of the mons veneris and lower abdominal wall by skin expansion as the last stage of surgical treatment of bladder exstrophy. Plast Reconstr Surg 1993; 91: 551–555

28. Audry G, Grapin C, Loulidi S et al. Penile reconstruction in exstophy. Ann Urol (Paris) 1991; 25: 120–124

29. Woodhourse C R J, Ransley P G, Williams D I. The patient with exstophy in adult life. Br J Urol 1983; 55: 632–635

30. King L R. The inadequate penis in some males with exstrophy — a plea for early sex conversion. Paper presented at the American Urological Association Annual Meeting, 1982: 116 (abstr 153)

31. Hanna M K, Williams D I. Genital function in males with vesical exstrophy and epispadias. Br J Urol 1972; 44: 169–174

31. Husmann D A, McClorie G A, Churchill B M. Phallic reconstruction in cloacal exstrophy. J Urol 1989; 142: 563–564

32. Davies J H A, Woodhouse C R J. Long term outcome of bladder exstrophy. Paper presented at the American Academy of Pediatrics, Washington, 1993, Abstr 50

33. Lattimer J K, Macfarlane M T, Puchor P J. Male exstrophy patients: a preliminary report on the reproductive capability. Trans Am Assoc Genito-Urin Surg 1979; 70: 42–46

34. Shapiro E, Lepor H, Jeffs R D. The inheritance of the exstrophy–epispadias complex. J Urol 1984; 132: 308–310

35. Blakeley C R, Mills W G. The obstetric and gynaecological complications of bladder exstrophy and epispadias. Br J Obstet Gynaecol 1981; 88: 167–173

36. Clemston C A B. Ectopia vesicae and split pelvis. J Obstet Gynaecol 1958; 65: 973–981

37. Krisiloff M, Puchner P J, Tretter W et al. Pregnancy in women with exstrophy. J Urol 1975; 119: 478–479

11

Urinary tract reconstruction in exstrophy and incontinent epispadias

S. Arap   A. M. Giron

Introduction and historical aspects

Before the 1960s, reconstructive surgery for bladder exstrophy was usually accompanied by high failure rates. Since the last century, several techniques have been described, which can be subdivided into three categories: (a) autoplastic flaps, aiming to cover the open anterior aspect of the bladder; (b) anatomical closure of the bladder, which constitutes the functional reconstruction, and (c) urinary diversions, with or without urinary bladder reconstruction.

Autoplastic flaps, obtained from adjacent skin or scrotum are composed of one or two layers. They have been used to cover the anterior portion of the bladder, protecting it from external irritation. However, surgical failure was almost universal, due to infection, devitalization of the flaps and the poor antiseptic armamentarium that existed at the time.[1,2]

Trendelenburg,[3] at the end of the last century, attempted to bring both pubic bones together, in the course of bladder reconstruction. On the basis of cadaveric studies, he proposed arthrotomy of the sacroiliac joint and medial rotation of the pubic bones. Patients were then immobilized in an orthopaedic device for 3–4 months, to allow a smooth osteosynthesis. Bladder reconstruction was performed simultaneously. This technique established the first hallmark in the treatment of bladder exstrophy, creating an iliac osteotomy.

Urinary incontinence was the major complication of this technique. Following these disappointing results, new methods were developed, such as urinary diversion into the rectum and sigmoid. Complete urinary continence and preservation of self-image were usually achieved, and several experimental and clinical studies were conducted. High incontinence rates and the risk of upper urinary tract dilation that usually occurred when attempts were made to preserve a functional bladder encouraged many authors to support urinary diversion.

Simon[4] was the first surgeon to divert the urinary stream to the large bowel in a patient with bladder exstrophy. Subsequently, in 1892, Maydl et al.[5] transposed the entire trigone and ureterovesical junctions, implanting them in the sigmoid colon. Using this technique, Gregoir and Schulman[6] reported excellent results in 72% of patients with regard to renal function, clinical condition and urinary continence, as well as good social adaptation.

Until the 1950s, ureterosigmoidostomy was the most popular diversion technique for treatment of bladder exstrophy. Techniques described by Coffey,[7] Leadbetter[8] and Goodwin et al.[9] were applied. Late complications such as stenosis of the ureterosigmoid anastomosis, pyelonephritis, hyperchloraemic acidosis and colon neoplasia precluded general acceptance of these techniques.[10–14] Rectal neobladder and ilial conduits were developed to avoid such complications. Goes[15,16] showed that a rectal neobladder offered a 66.6% rate of both urinary and faecal continence; the ileal conduit[17] is also associated with late complications such as pyelonephritis, urinary obstruction and chronic renal failure.

Hendren[18] utilized a modification of the ureterosigmoidostomy for bladder exstrophy, using a colon conduit as a temporary diversion. This conduit, often constructed in the first year of life, was then diverted 3–4 years later after ensuring that anal continence, antireflux mechanisms and renal function were adequate. This type of diversion is usually safer than those described above, although careful periodic evaluation of renal function is mandatory.

Parallel to the initial urinary diversions, Young,[19] in 1922, published a technique for treating incontinent epispadias; this technique consisted of 'narrowing' the bladder neck and posterior urethra. Dees and Durham,[20] in 1942, constructed a urethral tube involving the bladder neck and preserving the trigone. This technique, also known as Young–Dees, has been used extensively for the treatment of urinary incontinence due to exstrophy, epispadias, urogenital and sinus anomalies, and neuropathic bladder.[21–23]

Bladder exstrophy reconstruction, by constriction of the bladder neck and cystorrhaphy, is complicated by vesicoureteral reflux in approximately 90% of cases, followed by ureterohydronephrosis and renal damage. In a review article published in 1974, Johnston and Kogan[24] analysed primary reconstruction of bladder exstrophy by the Young–Dees technique, associated with osteotomy, and reported a urinary continence rate of 21.9%; however, there appeared to be no clear criteria for evaluation of continence and this rate was probably an overestimate. Continence was achieved, but uretherohydronephrosis was also common. Megali and Lattimer[25] reported various degrees of obstruction in 100% of cases.

In the authors' institution, comparable results were obtained using this technique from 1959 to 1965 for primary bladder exstrophy reconstruction: complete urinary continence and preservation of renal function was achieved in only one of 23 patients. The remaining 22 patients experienced complications such as small bladder capacity, vesicoureteral reflux and ureterohydronephrosis, a high incidence of urinary leaks, and re-exstrophy. The majority of patients (70%) ultimately required urinary diversion through either ileal conduits or rectal neobladders, as the ureteral dilatation almost always precluded ureterosigmoidostomy.[26]

Clinical presentation: description of the anomaly

These malformations occur in 1:30 000 to 1:50 000 live births, being twice as common in male as in female patients.[27,28]

Clinically, different signs can be detected and these variables bear a direct relation to successful reconstruction. The age of the child is important and the best results are obtained when treatment is initiated in the newborn. Early closure and protection of the bladder plate preserve the mucosa and preclude fibrosis and infection. The size and the characteristics of the exposed bladder vary: it may be an elastic, large bladder that is easily inverted manually (Fig. 11.1a, b); conversely, the bladder may be rigid and fibrotic, resisting invagination or reconstruction.

The bladder mucosa can be smooth and thin, with a soft muscular wall at birth, or congenital and/or acquired changes such as squamous,

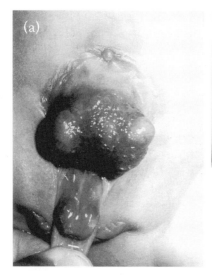
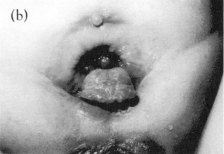

Figure 11.1. Bladder exstrophy suitable for reconstruction: (a) mucosa is thin; complete epispadias; bladder everted with abdominal pressure; (b) muscular bladder wall is elastic and can be inverted digitally.

glandular or polypoid metaplasia may be present. An associated inflammatory process can infiltrate the muscular layer and bladder plate will progressively lose its elasticity and become fibrotic and rigid. Most pathological changes can be prevented by early closure of the exstrophic bladder.[29,30] The umbilicus is attached cranial to the exstrophy.

The upper urinary tract is generally normal, even in untreated patients; a few patients may have renal agenesis or obstructive uropathy.

Pubic diastasis is the hallmark of the exstrophy–epispadias complex; it is smaller in epispadias and maximal in bladder and cloacal exstrophy, and is always associated with lateral rotation of the femur and acetabulum. The abdominal wall defect that remains after the bladder closure is triangular: it is limited laterally by the rectus abdominis muscle and inferiorly by the intersymphyseal fibrous band, which includes the external urinary sphincter. The perineal floor is compromised by the malformation, explaining the frequent occurrence of rectal prolapse; the anus lies anterior to its original site in both sexes.

Males present with an epispadic penis, short and wide at its base and dorsally curved; the urethra is represented by a dorsal strip of mucosa. The penile size is variable, but is usually small, imposing serious problems in obtaining an adequate phallus even after reconstruction. The scrotum is wide, and lack of testicular descent is common. True cryptorchidism is an uncommon associated anomaly. The testes are usually located at the external inguinal ring and can be manipulated into the scrotum. Inguinal hernias, probably related to a lateral abdominal fascial weakness, are more common and require repair.

The female typically has bifid clitoris; the internal genitalia are generally normal, but some cases will present with vaginal and uterine anomalies. The urethra also is epispadic and extremely short.

Exstrophic anomalies

Epispadias is the second most frequent anomaly and several variations occur, according to the position of the meatus — balanic, penile and penopubic in the male. It is a minor form of exstrophic complex and represents a rare anomaly, with an incidence of 1:117604 in male and 1:481110 in female patients.[27,28,30] The diagnosis is not easily made in females: the external characteristic — bifid clitoris — is visible only on careful examination of the genitalia (Figs 11.2–11.4).

Epispadias accounts for 30% of all exstrophic anomalies.

Cloacal exstrophy takes place when cloacal membrane dehiscence precedes urorectal septum formation. The median exstrophic plate is represented by exposed intestinal mucosa, generally the ileocaecal zone. Two bowel luminal orifices are seen, a superior (ileum) and an inferior

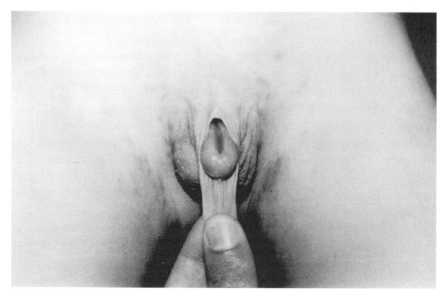

Figure 11.2. Penopubic incontinent epispadias in male.

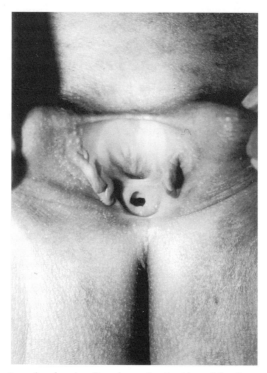

Figure 11.3. Incontinent female epispadias: the urethra is wide and the clitoris is bifid.

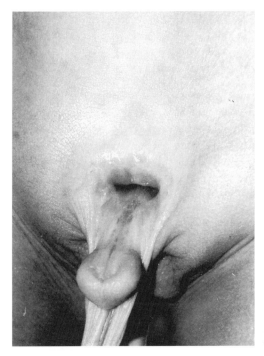

Figure 11.4. Intermediate type of exstrophy–epispadias.

(colonic remnant of the hindgut), that ends blindly in the pelvis. The lateral portions of the plate are made up of two hemibladders, each with its ureteral orifice. Prolapsed ileum and imperforate anus are almost always present. The appendix may open in the bowel exstrophy. The genitalia may take bizarre forms such as phallic duplication and scrotal ectopy. It is usually difficult to assign phenotypic sex.[31,32]

Duplicate exstrophy is associated with pubic diastasis. There are remnants of bladder mucosa at the abdominal wall surface, coexisting with a closed and integral bladder that may even be continent. It can coexist with complete epispadias or with a closed urethra in a stubby penis; pubic separation is always present and two of the authors' five cases were continent (three male and two female patients).

Superior vesical fissure is a small eventration of the bladder dome. The bladder and genitalia are otherwise normal, but pubic diastasis is present, distinguishing the lesion from a persistent urachus.

In *intestinal sequestration and exstrophy*, intestinal loops protrude with an inverted mucosa over the exstrophic elements but without any communication with the digestive tract, which is otherwise normal.

Pseudo-exstrophy or *covered exstrophy* consists of separated pubic bones and divergent rectus muscles, delimiting a ventral defect that is occupied by a closed and complete bladder. The genital anomalies are minimal.[33]

Objectives of surgical reconstruction

The goals of surgical treatment of bladder exstrophy are to obtain a continent child with a normal upper urinary tract and an abdominogenital reconstruction that makes possible a normal sexual and social life. Treatment must be individualized and subjected to a careful and long-term follow-up by the urologist. The therapeutic strategy should be adapted (depending on several factors) to the progress of each patient: bladder plates that initially are very small may expand considerably and develop into an adequate bladder cavity; conversely, bladders that are initially very large and elastic may develop fibrosis and even become non-compliant, frequently leading to ureteral dilatation. In those cases where a functional capacity is not attained, bladder augmentation should be undertaken to obtain a satisfactory urinary reservoir. Finally, persistent incontinence will demand other alternatives, such as the construction of continent urinary reservoirs associated with intermittent catheterization or even the use of artificial sphincters.

Technical advances associated with current success

Recently, the best results have been attained in functional reconstruction, particularly when a staged approach is planned and carried out. Continence is achieved in nearly 70% of cases and renal function is preserved in the majority. These advances took three decades to achieve after the initial attempts at bladder closure, because of the only gradual increase in understanding of the pathophysiology of incontinence, of the mechanisms of continence and of vesicourethral function and of the importance of vesicoureteric reflux causing upper urinary deterioration, together with the advent of intermittent clean catheterization and the artificial urinary sphincter. Also very important was the development of ingenious techniques to correct reflux, and to correct incontinence utilizing the bladder wall and particularly the trigone, tubularized to create a structure with the form and function of a sphincter. Finally, the roles of bladder capacity and bladder compliance in allowing perfect continence are now well understood. Bladder augmentation,[34–36] particularly with a detubularized intestinal loop,[37] is a useful procedure in many cases.

Many urologists have contributed to these advances.[38–45] More recently, there has been further progress in genital reconstruction, and the concepts of penile elongation through the liberation of the crura from its bone insertions have been challenged.[46,47]

An ingenious and elegant procedure, termed the Cantwell–Ransley technique, enables a much better cosmetic appearance to be obtained, with correction of the penile curvature, facilitating urethral access for urological manipulation and endoscopy.[48]

Institutional experience

From 1955 to 1994, more than 300 cases of the bladder exstrophy–epispadias complex were dealt with at the Division of Urology, Hospital das Clinicas, Faculdade de Medicina, Universidade de São Paulo. Table 11.1 lists the various types of exstrophic anomalies that were treated. Table 11.2 summarizes the alternative surgical treatments offered to these patients. Until 1963, urinary diversions using an ileal

Anomaly	No. of cases
Classical bladder exstrophy	221
Epispadias	58
Cloacal exstrophy	7
Intermediate forms of exstrophy–epispadias	5
Duplicate exstrophy	4
Superior vesical fissure	2
Exstrophy and intestinal sequestration	4
Total	301

Table 11.1. Types of exstrophic anomaly receiving treatment in the authors' institution between 1955 and 1994

Procedure	No. of cases
Functional primary reconstruction	27
Ileal conduit (Bricker)	23
Colonic conduit	5
Neorectal bladder	11
Colocystoplasty (Arap procedure)	29
Ureterosigmoidostomy, transcolonic conduit	19
Enterocystoplasty	9
Staged reconstruction of bladder exstrophy	88
Young–Dees–Leadbetter (epispadias)	22
Tanagho's procedure (epispadias)	18
Total	251

Table 11.2. Procedures for reconstruction of vesical exstrophy and epispadias

conduit and/or neorectal bladder were the commonest form of treatment. However, poor preservation of renal function, quality of life, metabolic stability of the patients, and even poor continence (in those with rectal neobladders) prompted a trial of functional reconstruction, based on the Young–Dees procedure.

Up to 1968, 27 patients were submitted to functional single-stage reconstruction; follow-up was possible in 21. Only one patient became fully continent; she developed good bladder capacity and no reflux, despite not having received vesicoureteroplasty. In all the remaining patients the treatment failed, leading to incontinence of varying degrees; ureterohydronephrosis, vesicoureteral reflux, stones, dehiscence of the bladder closure and urinary tract infection were common features postoperatively. For this reason, urinary diversions, particularly through ileal conduits, were made before bladder expansion could take place. In fact, bladder neck narrowing, associated with a small bladder and reflux, were fundamental factors leading to ureteral dilatation and hydronephrosis, thereby necessitating urinary diversion (and, simultaneously, precluding ureterosigmoidostomy as an alternative solution).

Since 1968, a programme designed to avoid the complications that arose in the single-stage functional reconstruction series has been initiated. Table 11.3 describes the possible complications of reconstructions, and the measures that can be taken to avoid such problems. Essentially, in a staged procedure, the aim was to attain a bladder of large volume and low pressure, into which the ureters would be implanted in an antireflux manner. Continence was provided through subtotal bladder tubularization, to which the large intestinal loop was anastomosed. This 'complete reconstruction of bladder exstrophy' led to improved continence rates associated with a higher rate of late morbidity. Reflux correction was very effective, through implantation of the ureters in the sigmoid colon[36–38] (Fig. 11.5).

Complication	Procedure
Small bladder capacity	Bladder augmentation
Fistulas and dehiscence	Dry reconstruction
Reflux	Ureteral reimplantation
Short penis	Penile elongation
Incontinence	Trigonal tubularization
Abdominal wall defect	Rotation of abdominal flaps

Table 11.3. Possible complications of bladder exstrophy reconstruction, and ways of overcoming them

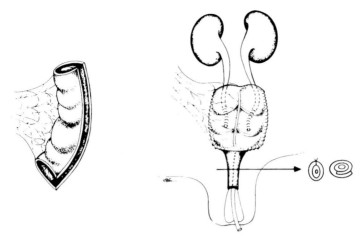

Figure 11.5. Arap procedure: a non-refluxing detubularized colonic conduit is anastomosed to a tubularized bladder tube.

Large bladder capacities with low intravesical pressures ensured upper urinary tract preservation; spontaneous voiding was frequently achieved, but many patients had to have recourse to clean intermittent catheterization in order to empty their bladders.

Late follow-up indicated that some initially small bladders developed to acceptable volumes, with the non-detubularized colonic loop attached to the bladder as a diverticulum (Fig. 11.6). Many patients presented with frequent small urinary losses due to intestinal contraction, as detected on urodynamic evaluation.

Concurrently, many publications, especially those by the Baltimore group,[49,50] have reported excellent results with the 'staged functional reconstruction' proposed by Fisher and Retik,[51] Cendron,[52] and Jeffs.[53]

Staged reconstruction — today

Since 1982, the authors have employed an individualized treatment, termed 'staged functional reconstruction'. Management is adapted to the clinical, urodynamic and radiological condition of each patient and is individualized throughout each step of the reconstruction process.[54–56]

Staged functional reconstruction consists of three surgical steps, as outlined below.

First stage
Vesical closure is performed without attempting to achieve continence; bladder exstrophy is then converted to incontinent epispadias. In the

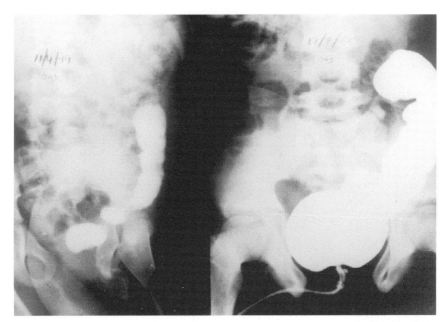

Figure 11.6. Non-detubularized colocystoplasty (initial Arap procedure); a small bladder (left) can attain a large capacity after years (right), even after subtotal bladder plate tubularization.

same procedure, penile elongation and abdominal wall reconstruction are performed, complemented by hernial repair and orchiopexy, when necessary (Fig. 11.7).

The objectives of this procedure are to protect the bladder mucosa and to prevent infection, metaplastic change and detrusor fibrosis, simultaneously allowing the bladder to develop its functional capacity. Experience has shown that, although incontinence exists, in 2–3 years the bladder may attain a functional capacity of 50–60 ml, which is the minimum volume necessary for the second surgical step (Fig. 11.8). Bladder closure may be associated with iliac osteotomy to facilitate pubic approximation; however, this is less commonly used in neonates. The authors advocate abdominal wall closure with the use of flaps, as described below. Although osteotomy is effective for this purpose, an equally efficient result can be obtained without its potential complications.

Osteotomy

In older children, iliac or innominate osteotomy are advocated to facilitate the abdominal wall closure through pubic approximation. The symphysis pubis usually spreads again, and the appearance on radiological examination is similar to the preoperative one. Whether pubic

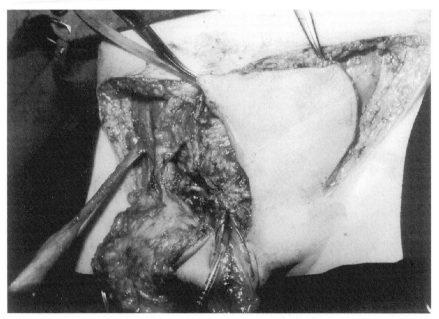

Figure 11.7. Staged reconstruction, first stage: penile elongation, cystorraphy and rotation of abdominal flaps, without osteotomy; hernial repair and orchiopexy.

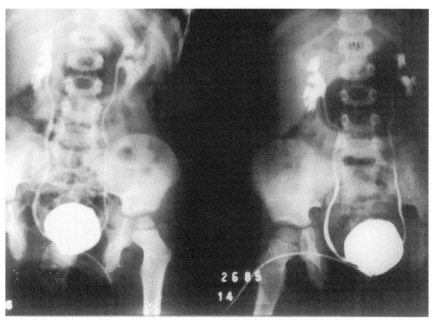

Figure 11.8. Cystography after the first stage; the vesicoureteral reflux is common and the bladder capacity will be evaluated.

approximation is important for urinary control, as Jeffs[53] and Chisholm[57] believe, or is helpful only in abdominal wall closure, is a controversial issue. The authors' opinion is that osteotomy is not crucial in attaining continence; furthermore, some authors believe that it causes additional shortening of the penis. The present authors close the abdominal wall defect through rotation of cutaneous and fascial flaps, with gratifying results: the cosmetic result is excellent, solid support is offered to the closed bladder, and the procedure is less time consuming and less traumatic for the child.

Several techniques have been described for osteotomy. Schultz,[58] in 1958, reintroduced posterior pelvic osteotomy when functional reconstruction of the vesical exstrophy was attempted. He concluded, in 1960, that the procedure is ideal, providing a satisfactory repair of the orthopaedic defect permitting bladder reconstruction, and positioning it in its habitual pelvic location. An interval of 1 week is allowed between osteotomy and cystorrhaphy; patients remain in a pelviopodalic (pelvis–feet) plaster cast for 60 days. The authors have utilized this procedure in their initial 40 cases.

Salter,[59] in 1961, described anterior osteotomy of the innominate bones, initially to correct congenital luxation and subluxation of the hip. The authors combined this procedure with vesical exstrophy reconstruction in seven patients; there was an interval of 7 days between osteotomy and exstrophy closure, and a pelviopodalic plaster cast was kept in place for approximately 30 days. The period of enforced immobility, the hospitalization period and the incidence of surgical infection were significantly lower than with posterior iliac osteotomy.

The authors conclude that osteotomy is an efficient method of closure of the abdominal wall as an auxiliary procedure, facilitating vesical reconstruction and reducing tissue tension. However, it is associated with a succession of drawbacks: it constitutes an additional surgical procedure; it calls for prolonged hospitalization; it promotes additional penile retraction, and the pelviopodalic plaster cast predisposes to infection, urinary fistula and bladder re-exstrophy.[60.]

Penile elongation is obtained with partial detachment of the crura from their ischial insertions and proximal detachment of the corpora cavernosa from the urethral strip, which improves dorsal chordee. Penile elongation is facilitated by the use of para-exstrophic skin, as described by Duckett.[61] Two flaps of this skin, which lies between the mucosa and the dermis, are outlined lateral to the bladder plate, remaining attached to the urethral strip. After penile elongation, these flaps are incorporated between the urethral strip and the prostatic apex, covering the additional penile length that has been developed. Liberating the crura from their bone attachments is currently a controversial issue, because some are of the opinion that this does not elongate the penile shaft; however, it is useful in preventing dorsal curvature.

After bladder closure, the authors drain the bladder through a urethral catheter; less commonly, ureteral stents, are used, particularly when the bladder is too small or when the mucosa is extremely hypertrophied. Redundant bladder polyps are usually resected to allow easier vesical closure.

Abdominoplasty (closure of the abdominal wall defect) is established by medial rotation of hypogastric flaps, including skin and the aponeuroses of the rectus and external oblique muscles. This procedure offers several advantages over osteotomy: it promotes reconstruction of the mons pubis with medial displacement of the hair-bearing skin; the reconstructed abdominal wall is quite strong and it does not retract the penis, as is ultimately the case with osteotomy. Frequently, hernia repair and/or orchiopexy are performed simultaneously (Figs 11.9 and 11.10). Postoperative hospitalization is short, usually 8–10 days. Although many authors believe that osteotomy helps to achieve continence through the approximation of the pelvic muscular floor around the urethra, this is certainly not an essential factor, as the present authors' results in relation

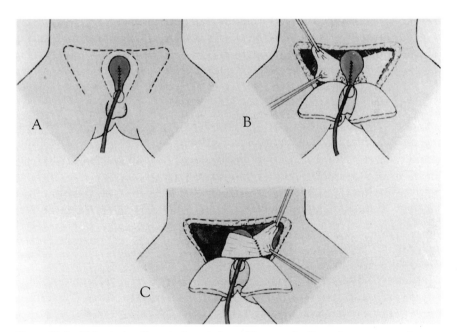

Figure 11.9. Abdominal wall repair through flaps of hypogastric skin and aponeuroses of rectus abdominis and external oblique muscles. (AUA Updated Series, Lesson 25, volume X, with permission of AUA Office of Education.)

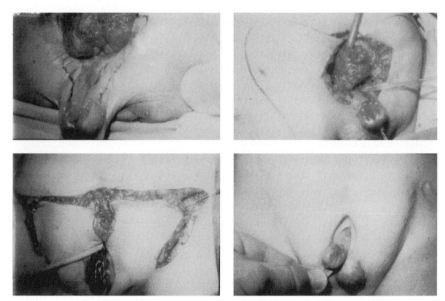

Figure 11.10. Surgical steps: exstrophy is closed to form an incontinent epispadias. The late result of abdominoplasty is shown at the lower right.

to continence are similar; additionally, the incidence of infections, fistulas, or dehiscence of the closure is very low.[62]

Umbilicoplasty is performed in this first stage of reconstruction; in the newborn the umbilical scar is medially relocated in the abdomen, at the level of the iliac crest. In older children omphaloplasty is performed by one of several techniques[63,64] (Fig. 11.11).

Initial bladder closure is indicated whenever bladder size and elasticity are adequate. This may be evaluated by inverting the bladder by digital manipulation or as demonstrated by its eversion when the child is crying (Fig. 11.1a, b). Some bladder plates that appear rigid may demonstrate the possibility of inversion under sedation. The authors tend to perform a closure in most cases. Bladders that, on presentation, initially had a volume of only 5–10 ml, have adequately expanded to 50 ml or more with time, permitting trigonal tubularization.

Whenever possible, this initial step is performed soon after birth in the first 7–10 days of life. An advantage of early closure is that the elasticity of the pelvic bones makes possible the approximation and primary reconstruction of the abdominal wall without having to perform osteotomy or to construct flaps.

The first surgical stage must be followed by careful examination for bacteriuria, monitoring the upper urinary tract with ultrasonographic evaluation, and an annual measurement of bladder functional capacity

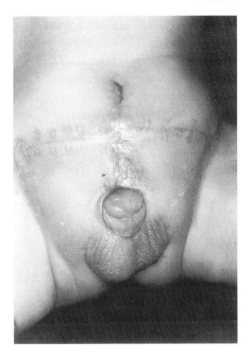

Figure 11.11. Abdominoplasty with omphaloplasty. (AUA Updated Series, Lesson 25, volume X, with permission of AUA Office of Education.)

by cystography. The second stage, as mentioned earlier, is performed when the minimal volume of 50 ml is attained.

Second stage

This step consists of bladder trigonal reconstruction to prevent vesicoureteric reflux and to provide continence through the Young–Dees–Leadbetter procedure.[8,20,23] It is the initial step in cases of epispadias, whenever bladder capacity is adequate.

A midline vertical incision is made through the reconstructed abdominal wall. The bladder is opened and a Cohen-type[65] bilateral ureteral reimplant is performed, relocating cranially the intravesical ureters and ureteral orifices. The trigone, liberated from the ureters, is incised bilaterally, delineating a median vertical rectangle of 2 × 5 cm, consisting of detrusor and overlying mucosa. The fundamental basis of this surgical procedure is to make a narrow strip of mucosa that can be tubularized over a number 4 or 6 feeding tube. The detrusor is then closed in an overlapping fashion. Vesical drainage is accomplished through a cystostomy, but a urethral catheter is left indwelling with a 'guideline' attached to its tip, which is exteriorized through the bladder and abdominal wall.

Ureteral catheters are left for 7–8 days, and urethral drainage is maintained for 10 days. The guideline is maintained to allow for planned urethral dilatation. Following removal of the urethral catheter, the cystostomy is clamped and voiding is stimulated. If urinary retention occurs, the guideline is used to dilate the urethra progressively until micturition ensues. The cystostomy also allows evaluation of residual urine after micturition, and it is removed when bladder emptying is adequate.

When urinary retention persists, endoscopy may eventually disclose obstructive mucosal folds, which can be incised very carefully.

Following bladder trigonal reconstruction, the child usually becomes continent after a period of several months. Continence is initially limited to short periods and improves as bladder capacity increases. Frequency and urgency are usually associated with the early postoperative period and persist until bladder capacity is adequate.

Third stage

Urethral reconstruction is performed usually after the anti-incontinence Leadbetter procedure. When bladder volume does not develop adequately, urethral tubularization adds resistance to bladder emptying, thereby further developing the bladder. In such cases, reconstruction can precede and facilitate the anti-incontinence procedure.

Several techniques have been proposed for urethroplasty,[66–69] but tubularizing the dorsal skin, as an inverted Duplay urethroplasty, has been the most popular procedure since proposed by Young.[69] Alternatively, the authors are currently using the Cantwell–Ransley technique.[48] The reconstruction includes wide mobilization of the ventral plate nourished by a mesentery of penoscrotal skin; the suspensory ligaments are divided and the corpora are detached from the pubis; urethral and glandular tubularization is then performed. Finally, the authors carry out chordee correction and penile skin coverage. The cosmetic penile aspect is satisfactory.

A commonly neglected technical aspect should be remembered when undertaking glandular reconstruction. Usually, a very thick glandular ventral aspect exists, which does not allow positioning of the urethral meatus at the tip of the penis, and the urethra opens at the dorsal aspect of the glans. It has been the authors' policy to initiate glandular reconstruction by a generous ventral incision at the midline, thus liberating distal glans tissue to be sutured over the urethra. The urethral meatus is positioned at the ventral aspect of the glans extremity. The glans is than denuded with scissors at its dorsal angle, bilaterally. The two parallel inner borders are sutured into a tubular urethra, the meatus of which will be the ventral incision previously performed. The two lateral borders are also sutured over the tubularized urethra, enabling cosmetically optimal glandular reconstruction.

In girls, clitoral reconstruction and subsequent enlargement of the vaginal introitus may be performed.

Results

Epispadias

A total of 48 children with incontinent epispadias (35 boys and 13 girls, aged 7 months to 15 years at the beginning of treatment) were treated between 1967 and 1994 with a follow-up of 5 months to 24 years. All patients presented with penopubic epispadias, except for three who presented with transitional forms between bladder exstrophy and epispadias. In all patients, bladder capacity was evaluated before operation. Reflux was present in 33% of cases.[70]

Forty-seven patients underwent suprapubic reconstruction of the bladder neck. Vesicoplasty was performed either by trigonal bladder tubularization (nine Young–Dees and 30 Leadbetter procedures) or by anterior bladder wall tubularization (eight Tanagho procedures). Of the three patients with minimal bladder capacity, one was treated by Arap's procedure[37] and two underwent minor constriction of the bladder neck to improve urinary retention and, consequently, bladder capacity and tonus; a secondary Leadbetter procedure was performed in both these patients.

Continence was achieved in 34 patients after the initial anti-incontinence operation, including 28 who maintained an excellent result during the initial 12–24 months of follow-up. All of these patients were older than 5 years, except for a 3-year-old boy. The remaining three patients acquired urinary control after longer periods and, coincidentally, they were the youngest children in the series (1, 2 and 3 years old). The establishment of continence had no relationship to puberty and in three cases continence preceded puberty. Generally, continence was preceded by a period of incomplete control during which longer dry periods between micturition were noted progressively. All children who became continent had been previously partially continent.

The results were similar for the three techniques (Table 11.4).

Bladder exstrophy

In the authors' institution, 88 patients with classical bladder exstrophy have been treated by means of the staged approach; 31 underwent bladder neck reconstruction by Young–Dees–Leadbetter technique (26 male and 5 female patients). Their ages at the second stage ranged from $2^1/_2$ to 17 years; the median follow-up time was 7 years. At this stage, the functional bladder capacity was over 50 ml. The remaining 57 patients are awaiting improvement in bladder capacity or have received treatment by other procedures (diversion, continent reservoir, etc.).

No. of patients	Leadbetter	Young–Dees	Tanagho	Total
Total	30	9	8	47 (100)*
Continent	22	7	5	34 (72.3)
Incontinent	8	2	3	13 (27.7)
With complications				
Ureterovesical obstruction	4	-	-	4 (8.5)
Reflux	5	4	3	12 (25.5)
Transient reflux	-	-	3	3 (6.4)
Bladder stones	-	-	3	3 (6.4)

*Percentages in parentheses.

Table 11.4. Epispadias repair: procedure, complications and results

Neonatal cystorrhaphy was achieved in 12 children, without abdominal flaps.

After the first step (cystorrhaphy), three patients underwent constriction of the bladder neck; this manoeuvre was useful to improve bladder capacity.

The 22 patients who achieved continence (70.9%) subsequently have not required any protection or nappies (diapers); three patients with enterocystoplasty are continent with intermittent self-catheterization. The four partially continent patients (13%) present stress incontinence, although they remain dry for periods of 1–2 h after voiding. The remaining five patients (16.1%) are incontinent; one of these underwent another Young–Dees–Leadbetter procedure and incontinence is secondary to poor bladder compliance in two (Table 11.5).

Urinary retention
In nine of the 31 patients (29%), acute urinary retention occurred when spontaneous micturition was attempted; intermittent bladder catheterization as well as urethral dilatation were required and in most cases the retention resolved without any auxiliary procedure.

Urodynamic evaluation
Urodynamic evaluation was carried out in only 16 patients, because of difficulty in catheterization in the remaining patients. Of these 16 patients, ten had urethrotrigonal outlet resistance with a urethral pressure profile of 89.3 cmH_2O over a length of 2.6 cm. Bladder compliance was compromised in 16 patients of the study, to varying

Continence	No. of patients
Continent	22 (70.9)*
(with intermittent catheterization)	(3)
Partially continent	4 (13.0)
Incontinent	5 (16.1)
Total	31 (100)

*Percentages in parentheses.

Table 11.5. Urinary continence in 31 patients after undergoing Young–Dees–Leadbetter bladder neck reconstruction

degrees; three of these have subsequently been submitted to enterocystoplasty.

Complications

Reflux was noted in nine (unilateral) ureteral units; in three patients this was corrected by transureteroureterostomy, to avoid additional bladder fibrosis.

Ureterovesical obstruction with ureterohydronephrosis occurred in two patients (no patient required nephrectomy and the renal function was preserved in all patients); three children had bladder stones.

Four patients had difficulty in emptying the bladder because of obstruction in the urethrotrigonal tube. They were treated with urethral dilatation, or urethrotomy under careful visual inspection.

Urethrocutaneous fistulas were noted in four patients; these were corrected by bladder drainage.

Finally, surgical results in epispadias and bladder exstrophy are very similar, with 70–75% of patients achieving continence and upper urinary tract preservation. Staged reconstruction, converting exstrophy into incontinent epispadias and allowing the development of adequate bladder capacity, makes both groups equal in terms of subsequent continence.

It should also be stressed that bladder exstrophy presents uniformly with marginally compromised bladder compliance, which, of course, deteriorates further on repeated surgery. Thus poorer results are achieved in those patients who have undergone previous surgery; it is essential that such patients are referred to centres specializing in surgical reconstruction.

Therapeutic algorithm

Staged functional reconstruction is currently almost always the initial treatment of choice (Fig. 11.12). Very rarely is urinary diversion, such as ureterosigmoidostomy, proposed for even the worst cases, with small and inelastic bladder plates. In such cases, total bladder tubularization associated with bladder substitution with intestine may be used as an alternative.[36]

Following the first stage, several scenarios are possible, as follows.

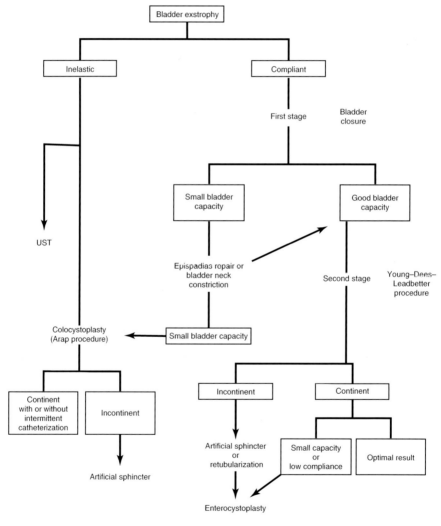

Figure 11.12. Therapeutic algorithm. (AUA Updated Series, Lesson 25, volume X, with permission of AUA Office of Education.)

Small bladder capacity

After closure of the bladder, two conditions may be present. Occasionally, where there are fibrotic bladder plates or in patients who have undergone reoperation, the bladder does not achieve the acceptable functional capacity essential for bladder trigonal reconstruction. In such cases, either by closing the epispadias or through constriction of the bladder neck, urethral resistance may be increased and additional expansion of the bladder volume may be obtained (Fig. 11.13). As in cases of epispadias with a small bladder, in which the results of an anti-incontinence procedure are very poor,[71] any manoeuvre that increases urethral resistance may lead to increased bladder functional capacity, allowing successful secondary trigonal tubularization.[38]

This small increase in urethral resistance, associated with tightening of the bladder neck or urethroplasty, may increase the bladder capacity, but may also increase intravesical pressure. Follow-up in this case must be very careful, in order to detect any damage to the upper urinary tract. In such situations, urethral dilatation may again provide adequate bladder emptying.

Occasionally, even after these alternative procedures, the bladder will not enlarge sufficiently. In this case, a long tube of detrusor is made to provide continence for colocystoplasty.[36] Currently, a detubularized intestinal segment (ileal, sigmoid or ileocaecal) is employed to obtain a continent reservoir that is drained through the urethra. Patients may

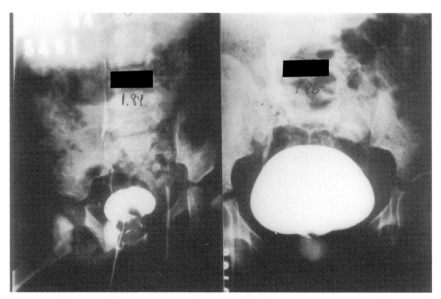

Figure 11.13. Small bladder after the first stage, 30 ml (left); constriction of bladder neck (right), and increased bladder capacity (100 ml) 2 years later.

become continent with or without intermittent catheterization; in those few cases in which incontinence persists, an artificial sphincter may give a satisfactory result.

Adequate bladder capacity

Whenever a bladder volume above 50 ml is attained, an anti-incontinence procedure is performed. These patients can usually be categorized into two groups. Patients in the first group are those with satisfactory urinary continence, allowing normal social behaviour, usually after several months of follow-up. Most of the authors' patients (60% as a rule), belong to this category, with urodynamic demonstration of almost normal bladder function and normal social continence. Patients in the second group have satisfactory sphincteric continence: they will remain dry for short periods, but are forced to empty their bladders every hour. Another subgroup comprises those patients who are continent for longer periods but in whom upper urinary tract dilatation is present; this is related to a poorly compliant bladder, either congenital or secondary to detrusor fibrosis.

As a rule, the functional capacity of reconstructed exstrophic bladders is smaller than usual, but the compliance may be normal or near normal. Occasionally, reduced bladder compliance limits continence and induces upper ureteral dilatation. The only solution for these patients is bladder augmentation with intermittent catheterization to empty the bladder. For those patients with continence and good bladder compliance, but in whom frequent voiding is necessary, a long period of follow-up should be provided and bladder augmentation used only as a last resort. For those patients with persistent urinary incontinence, bladder neck retubularization may be used but an artificial urinary sphincter may be indicated.

Urinary diversion represents the final alternative for those patients in whom all the previously described therapeutic modalities have failed. Ureterosigmoidostomy or a continent urinary diversion may represent the only acceptable solution in difficult cases of bladder exstrophy. This procedure, however, is seldom employed today.

Conclusions

Treatment of bladder exstrophy represents an example of how persistence and surgical ingenuity can improve results in reconstructive urinary surgery. Each patient must receive an individualized and personal follow-up, with careful evaluation of radiological, clinical and urodynamic data to plan the subsequent stages of reconstruction.

Finally, it must be stressed that success in urinary tract reconstruction is directly related to surgical experience: such patients should undergo surgery at centres where experienced and trained surgeons are available. Those urologists and surgeons that receive one such case every two or three years should refer them to specialized centres, thus offering them a greater chance of attaining a normal social and physiological life. Nevertheless, even in specialized centres, the success rate is much greater in primary 'virgin' cases than in those in which surgery has been performed previously.[45]

References

1. Orlow L. Traitement operatoire de l'exstrophie de la vessie: transplantation des uretères par le procédé de Maydl. Rev Gynécol 1903; 7: 795–852

2. O'Donnell B. The lessons of 40 bladder exstrophies in 20 years. J Pediatr Surg 1984; 19: 547–549

3. Trendelenburg F. The treatment of ectopia vesicae. Ann Surg 1906; 44: 281–289

4. Simon J. Extopia vesicae: operation for diverting the orifices of the ureters into the rectum: temporary success; subsequent death; autopsy. Lancet 1850; 2: 568. Cited in Murphy L J T. Exstrophy of the bladder. In: Murphy L J T (ed) The history of urology. Springfield, Thomas, 1972: 333–377

5. Maydl K. Uber die Radikaltherapie der Extopia vesicae urinaire. Wien med Wschr 1894; 44: 1113–1169, 1209, 1256, 1297. Cited in Murphy L J T. Exstrophy of the bladder. In: Murphy L J T (ed) The history of urology. Springfield, Thomas, 1972: 333–377

6. Gregoir W, Schulman C C. Exstrophy of the bladder: treatment by trigonosigmoidostomy — long-term results. Br J Urol 1978; 50: 90–94

7. Coffey R C. Transplantation of the ureter into the large intestine in the absence of a functioning bladder. Surg Gynecol Obstet 1921; 32: 383–391

8. Leadbetter G W Jr. Surgical correction of total urinary incontinence. J Urol 1964; 91: 261–266

9. Goodwin W E, Harris A P, Kaufman J J. Open transcolonic ureterointestinal anastomosis. Surg Gynecol Obstet 1953; 97: 295–300

10. Lasser A, Acosta A E. Colonic neoplasms complicating ureterosigmoidostomy. Cancer 1975; 35: 1218–1222

11. Leadbetter G W Jr. Ureterosigmoidostomy and carcinoma of the colon. J Urol 1979; 121: 732–735

12. Megalli M, Lattimer J K. Review of the management of 140 cases of exstrophy of the bladder. J Urol 1973; 109: 246–248

13. Segura J W, Kelalis P D. Long term results of ureterosigmoidostomy in children with bladder exstrophy. J Urol 1975; 114: 138–140

14. Arap S. Ureterosigmoidostomy. In: Glenn J F (ed) Urologic surgery, 4th ed. Philadelphia: Lippincott, 1991: 1031–1036

15. Góes G M. Contribuição para o estudo da neobexiga retal. Tese (Doutorado), Faculdade dé Medicina, Universidade de São Paulo, São Paulo, 1969

16. Góes G M. Contribuição para o estudo da anastomose uretero-ileo-cutânea. Faculdada de Medicina Universidadae de São Paulo, Tese (Livre Docência), São Paulo, 1972

17. Campos Freire J G. Bricker operation in children. Urol Int 1968; 23: 89–93

18. Hendren H W. Exstrophy of the bladder. An alternative method of management. J Urol 1976; 115: 195–202
19. Young H H. A new operation for the cure of the incontinence associated with epispadias. J Urol 1922; 7: 1–32
20. Dees J E, Durham N C. Epispadias with incontinence in the male. Surgery 1942; 12: 621–630
21. Goldwasser R, Barret D M, Wein A J. Surgery of the neuropathic bladder. In: Libertino J A (ed) Pediatric and adult reconstructive urological surgery, 2nd ed. Baltimore: Williams and Wilkins, 1987; 419–443
22. Kramer S A, Kelalis P P. Correction of total incontinence in male and female epispadias. J Pediatr Surg 1981; 16: 812–815
23. Young H H. Exstrophy of the bladder. The first case in which a normal bladder and urinary control have been obtained by plastic operations. Surg Gynecol Obstet 1942; 74: 729–737
24. Johnston J H, Kogan S J. The exstrophic anomalies and their surgical reconstruction. In: Johnston J H, Kogan S J (eds) Current problems in surgery. Chicago: Year Book Medical, 1974: 1–39
25. Megalli M, Lattimer J K. Review of the management of 140 cases of exstrophy of the bladder. J Urol 1973; 109: 246–248
26. Arap S, Gonçalves E S, Gutierrez E G, Góes G M. Tratamento da extroifia de bexiga. I. Reconstrução plástica. AMB Rev Assoc Med Bras 1976; 22: 61–64
27. Higgins C C. Exstrophy of the bladder: report of the 158 cases. Ann Surg 1962; 28: 99–102
28. Rickham P P. The incidence and treatment of ectopia vesicae. Proc R Soc Med 1961; 54: 389–392
29. Rudin L, Tannenbaum M, Lattimer J K. Histologic analysis of the exstrophied bladder after anatomical closure. J Urol 1972; 108: 802–807
30. Johnston J H, Kogan S J. The exstrophic anomalies and their surgical reconstruction. In: Johnston J H, Kogan S J (eds) Current problems in surgery. Chicago: Year Book Medical, 1974: 1
31. Muecke E C. Exstrophy, epispadias and other anomalies of the bladder. In: Walsh P C, Guittes R F, Perlmutter A D, Stamey T A (eds) Campbell's Urology, 5th ed. Philadelphia: Saunders, 1986: 1856–1880
32. Johnston J H. The exstrophic anomalies. In: Williams D I, Johnston J H (eds) Peadiatric urology, 2nd ed. London: Butterworths, 1982: 299–316
33. Johnston J H, Koff S A. Covered cloacal exstrophy another variation on the theme. J Urol 1977; 118: 666–668
34. Couvelaire R, Moulonguet A, Sagot A. Sur le traitment de l'exstrophie vésicale. J Urol Nephrol 1961; 65: 757–782
35. Martinez-Pinero T A. Long term results of surgical treatment of bladder exstrophy. Eur Urol 1976; 2: 168–174
36. Arap S, Giron A M, Góes G M. Initial results of the complete reconstruction of bladder exstrophy. Urol Clin North Am 1980; 7: 477–491
37. Arap S, Giron A M, Góes G M. Staged reconstruction for bladder exstrophy using colonic conduits. In: Carlton C E Jr (ed) Controversies in urology. Chicago: Year Book Medical, 1988: 20–23
38. Arap S, Giron A M, Abrão E G et al. Nonrefluxing colonic conduit. Eur Urol 1980; 8: 196–200
39. Gearhart J P, Jeffs R D. Bladder exstrophy: increase in capacity following epispadias repair. J Urol 1989; 142: 525–526

40. Caione P, Capozza N, Lais A et al. Female genito-urethroplasty and submucosal periurethral collagen injection as adjunctive procedures for continence in the exstrophy-epispadias complex: preliminary results. Br J Urol 1993; 71: 350–353

41. Canning D A, Gearhart J P, Peppas D S, Jeffs R D. The cephalotrigonal reimplant in bladder neck reconstruction for patients with exstrophy or epispadias. J Urol 1993; 150: 156–158

42. Tanagho E A, Smith D R, Meyers F H, Fisher R. Mechanism of urinary continence. III. Technique for surgical correction of incontinence. J Urol 1969; 101: 305–316

43. Gibbon A J, Maffulli N, Fixsen J A. Horizontal pelvic osteotomies for bladder exstrophy. J Bone Joint Surg (Br) 1991; 73-B: 896–898

44. Hollowell J G, Hill P D, Duffy P G, Ransley P G. Bladder function and dysfunction in exstrophy and epispadias. Lancet 1991; 338: 926–928

45. Merguerian P A, McLorie G A, McMullin N D et al. Continence in bladder exstrophy: determinants of success. J Urol 1991; 145: 350–352

46. Thomala J V, Mitchell M E. Ventral prepucial island flap technique for repair of epispadias with or without exstrophy. J Urol 1984; 132: 985–987

47. Queiroz e Silva F A, Giron A M, Arap S. Balanoplastia no complexo epispadia–extrofia. J Bras Urol 1986; 12: 83–84

48. Ransley P G, Duffy P G, Wollin M. Bladder exstrophy closure and epispadias repair. In: Spitz L, Nixon H H (eds) Paediatric surgery. London: Butterworths, 1988; 620–632

49. Jeffs R D, Guide S L, Oesch I. The factors in successful exstrophy closure. J Urol 1982; 127: 974–976

50. Gearhart J P, Canning D A, Jeffs R D. Failed bladder neck reconstruction: options for management. J Urol 1991; 146: 1082–1084

51. Fisher J H, Retik A B. Exstrophy of the bladder. J Pediatr Surg 1969; 4: 620–627

52. Cendron J. La reconstruction vésicale. Méthode dérivée de celle de Trendelenburg. Ann Chir Infant 1971; 12: 371–390

53. Jeffs R D. Exstrophy. In: Harrison J H, Guittes R F, Perlmutter A D, Stamey T A (eds) Campbell's Urology, 4th ed, vol 2. Philadelphia: Saunders, 1979: 1672–1696

54. Arap S, Giron A M. Bladder exstrophy. In: Retik A B, Cukier J (eds) International perspectives in urology: pediatric urology. Baltimore: Williams and Wilkins, 1987: 282

55. Arap S, Giron A M. Bladder exstrophy: reconstructive alternatives. AUA Update Series 1991; Lesson 25, vol X: 194–200

56. Arap S, Giron A M. Bladder exstrophy: epispadias. In: Krane R J, Siroky M B, Fitzpatrick J M (eds) Clinical urology. Philadelphia: Lippincott, 1994; 786–797

57. Chisholm T C. Exstrophy of the urinary bladder. Am J Surg 1961; 101: 649–655

58. Shultz W C. Plastic repair of exstrophy of bladder combined with bilateral osteotomy of ilia. J Urol 1958; 7: 453–458

59. Salter R B. Innominate osteotomy in the treatment of the congenital dislocation and subluxation of the hip. J Bone Joint Surg (Am) 1961; 43-A: 518–539

60. Giron A M, Arap S, Góes G M. Experiência com a osteotomia pélvica na reconstrução cirúrgica da extrofia vesical. Rev Hosp Clin Fac Med São Paulo 1984; 39: 107–112

61 Duckett J W. The use of paraexstrophy skin pedicle grafts for correction of exstrophy and epispadias repair. Birth Defects 1977; 13: 171–175

62. Giron A M. Reparação da parede abdominal em extrofia vesical, por meio de retalhos cutâneos hipogástricos compostos e simples. Tese (Doutorado), Faculdade de Medicina da Universidade de São Paulo, São Paulo, 1987

63. Baroudi R. Umbilicoplasty. Clin Plast Surg 1975; 2: 431–448
64. Hanna M K, Asong K. Reconstructions of umbilicus in bladder exstrophy. Urology 1978; 24: 324–326
65. Cohen S J. The Cohen reimplantation technique. Birth Defects 1977; 13: 391–395
66. Johnston J H. Epispadias. In: Harrison J H, Guittes R J, Perlmutter A D (eds) Campbell's Urology, 4th ed. Philadelphia: Saunders, 1978; 1663–1697
67. Duckett J W. Epispadias. Urol Clin North Am 1978; 5: 107–126
68. Tanagho E A. Male epispadias: surgical repairs of urethropenile deformity. Br J Urol 1976; 48: 127–134
69. Young H H . A new operation for epispadias. J Urol 1918; 2: 237–243
70. Arap S, Nahas W C, Giron A M et al. Incontinent epispadias: surgical treatment of 38 cases. J Urol 1988; 140: 577–581
71. Klauber G T, Williams D I. Epispadias with incontinence. J Urol 1974; 111: 110–113

Reconstructive surgery of the lower genitourinary tract in children

12

R. Hohenfellner   R. Wammack

Introduction

Neurogenic disorders, congenital anomalies, iatrogenic lesions and malignancies represent the main indications for reconstructive urogenital surgery in childhood. The goal of this surgery is to restore the individual to normal. The question arises as to which operative strategy is most suited to achieve this goal and when this intervention should take place.

Adolescent patients and young adults in particular have definite expectations pertaining to the outcome of this surgery; voiding should be possible through the urethra under voluntary control, at convenient intervals and in the absence of urinary tract infections. Continence is of paramount importance, as it affects every aspect of social and professional life. The impact and implications of night-time incontinence are often overlooked: many authors remark merely that this problem might easily be solved by the use of a nappy (diaper) at night; however, the consequences in puberty and, later, in a partnership are extremely detrimental.

The patient's wishes, however, are not always in line with the urologist's concerns in planning reconstructive lower tract surgery. The procedure that is chosen must be adapted to the patient's mental capacity. A continent internal reservoir needs clean intermittent catheterization (CIC) at regular intervals and, in the first months after surgery, regular irrigation for mucus evacuation is necessary. These procedures, of course, call for a certain level of intelligence and responsibility in patients to ensure their compliance. Moreover, a patient's orthopaedic status is a decisive factor: for wheelchair-bound patients, urethral CIC is nearly impossible or is, to say the least, impractical; an almost invisible stoma located in the umbilical funnel is preferable.

Renal function often limits the number of possible alternative procedures. Continent diversion is preferable in many respects: nevertheless, this type of diversion may not be beneficial if renal function is severely compromised. Experience has shown that the borderline creatinine level is 1.5 mg/dl; if renal function is less efficient then continent urinary diversion is too risky.

Up to the point when the child enters school, urinary continence is not a major issue as the home and parents create a protective and understanding environment. With increasing social contact in school or at a friend's house, this aspect becomes crucial. With the onset of puberty, body image is very important.

Intermittent catheterization, antibiotic prophylaxis and anticholinergic drugs have significantly lowered the rate of parenchymal infection during the first years of life and have thus substantially improved the chances of subsequent urinary tract reconstruction. When the adolescent or young adult leaves the protective and supportive environment of the family home, compliance steadily decreases. These aspects must all be considered when planning reconstructive surgery in the child.

Therapeutic strategies

In order to stabilize renal function in an infection-free environment while permitting urinary continence, it is essential to assess correctly the limitations and risks of surgery. Despite all the progress in reconstructive surgery, a fully functional sphincter can not be constructed. All attempts in this direction represent merely 'balanced obstruction' and constitute a compromise with an unpredictable and, all too often, an unfavourable outcome. The higher the degree of obstruction, the more likely is a final condition with CIC; the more incomplete the obstruction, the more unsatisfactory the result, because a life with diapers is the consequence.

Artificial sphincters

Artificial sphincters are widely implemented to create continence but, in children in particular, the results of such a procedure give no cause for congratulations (Table 12.1).[1–6] Results in adults are not much better. In a series of 100 patients, Nurse and Mundy report a 45% complication rate.[7] Recently, a paper investigating children with the AMS 800 sphincter demonstrated that in 50% of cases silicone shedding occurred.[8] The long-term effects are entirely unknown. In the authors' opinion, artificial sphincters should not be implanted before puberty, because of the high rate of complications and the moderate success rate.

Bladder neck reconstruction

Bladder neck reconstruction (BNR) using the Young–Dees procedure or one of its many modifications have variable and often unsatisfactory

Author	No. of patients	Complication rate (%)	Continence rate (%)	Reference no.
Light	132	24	70	1
Gonzalez	15	38	67*	2
Aprilian	27	39	88	3
Bosco	36	61	74†	4
Grein	39	56	87	5
Barratt	45	60		6

*34% explanted; †25% explanted.

Table 12.1. Results of artificial sphincter implantation in children

results. Despite improvements in technique, 30–50% of patients remain incontinent and have many other voiding difficulties and complaints[9,10] (Fig. 12.1).[11] The present authors' results have been no better (Table 12.2). A recent review from the Indiana University Hospitals has demonstrated the damage that this procedure can also cause to the upper urinary tract (Table 12.3).[9] Only 57% of patients had normal imaging studies of the upper urinary tract after BNR. At least one surgeon has abandoned attempts of achieving continence using this technique and has gone on to perform bladder augmentation along with a suprapubic Mitrofanoff stoma for CIC (P. G. Ransley, personal communication). In view of the long-term results, much of the enthusiasm associated with BNR surgery in early publications has given way to scepticism. Although some centres still report that up to 80% of their patients achieve 'an excellent surgical result',[12,13] this is defined as one soiling per day and dry intervals of 3 h.

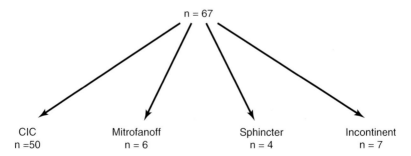

Figure 12.1. Results of bladder neck reconstruction and bladder augmentation in children with bladder exstrophy. CIC, clean intermittent catheterization. Data from ref. 11.

Outcome	No. of children
Complete continence	1
Daytime continence, partial night-time continence	2
Daytime continence, night-time incontinence	2
Complete incontinence	2[†]
No spontaneous voiding	1[†]

*Ages 3–13 years.
†Conversion.

Table 12.2. Results of Mainz pouch augmentation and modified Young–Dees procedure in eight children*

Outcome	Percentage of patients
Continence	39–64
Reoperation	27–75
Upper tract deterioration	24

*Source, ref. 9.

Table 12.3. Results of Young–Dees bladder neck reconstruction 1978–1988, in 47 patients*

In a large prospective urodynamic study comparing patients with closed exstrophied bladders before and after bladder neck reconstruction, Hollowell,[14–16] as well as Kazachkov,[17] have shown that incontinence is mainly due to bladder instability and is not solely a result of insufficient outlet resistance. The closed exstrophied bladder produces involuntary contractions that cause a substantial rise of intravesical pressure, which easily overcomes the leak point pressure. Neuropharmacological investigations by the authors have indicated that alterations in the innervation and neurophysiology of these exstrophied bladders are responsible for these observations. The lack of response of these bladders to anticholinergic therapy seems to be attributable to functional abnormalities of the cholinergic receptor and the presence of non-adrenergic-non-cholinergic innervation.

Management of continence
A substantial number of children have to perform CIC to evacuate their bladder or require CIC to be continent, at least to some degree. Data analysis has also shown that, for some reason, gender seems to have a

role: whereas those female patients with bladder exstrophy who are able to void without residual urine after bladder neck reconstruction have demonstrated a low complication rate, male patients have encountered significantly more problems.

The problem of producing continence is not specific to those with exstrophied bladder. Every form of incontinence is difficult to manage, especially in children. For practical purposes, a difference must be made between patients with a functioning sphincter (leak-point pressure > 25 cmH$_2$O) and a small bladder capacity (< 100 ml) and patients with an incompetent sphincter (leak-point pressure < 25 cmH$_2$O). The best results with bladder augmentation alone have been achieved when iatrogenic bladder lesion or neurogenic bladder with an outlet resistance of more than 25 cmH$_2$O was the indication for intervention. Such patients benefit from bladder augmentation alone particularly if they are not wheelchair-bound and even if spontaneous voiding is not possible and CIC is necessary. If the outlet resistance has to be increased, then sling plasties[18–20] seem to produce the most satisfactory results and are most certainly preferable to artificial sphincters (see also Chapter 22 of this volume).

In the authors' series of patients, the orthopaedic status was of major significance. Non-wheelchair-bound patients demonstrate less upper urinary tract damage, whereas wheelchair-bound patients show a tendency to gain weight as they become older and also experience increasing problems of continence during physical activity, which becomes evident during everyday activities such as getting into and out of a car. With increasing disproportion of the upper part of the body, the umbilicus moves towards the symphysis. Female patients showing such changes have particular difficulty in performing urethral CIC. For all of these patients the Mainz pouch I with a nearly 'invisible' umbilical stoma is the method of choice. This procedure yields beneficial results and produces a low rate of complications (Table 12.4).

Avoidance of complications

The last 10 years have provided many lessons on how to avoid certain complications. Obstruction at the site of ureterointestinal anastomosis was primarily seen in patients with preoperatively dilated upper urinary tracts. An extraperitoneal approach to the pouch from a right-sided flank incision has proved very beneficial for repair of ureterointestinal stricture (Fig. 12.2). After the pouch is opened (Fig. 12.3), the ureter is reimplanted by means of a short submucosal tunnel (Figs 12.4 and 12.5). When the pouch is of sufficient capacity, the risk of reflux is minimal. Stoma stenosis, a frequent problem in the authors' early series, is

Complication	Treatment	No. of complications
Early		
Ileus	Op. revision*	4
Pouch tamponade	Endoscopic evacuation	2
Wound dehiscence	Op. revision	2
Intestinal fistula	Conservative treatment	2
Nipple necrosis	New ileum nipple	1
Appendix necrosis	Ileum nipple	1
Spontaneous pouch rupture	Op. revision	1
		13/314 (4.1%)
Late		
Stones	Endoscopic treatment	27
Stomal stenosis	Endoscopic treatment	23
Ureteral stenosis	Neoimplantation	18
	Nephrectomy	5
Ileus	Op. revision*	4
Pouch perforation	Op. revision	3
Nipple gliding	Op. revision	3
Pouch tamponade (mucus)	Endoscopic treatment	2
Appendix stoma dislocation	Ileum nipple	1

*Operative revision in three patients.

Table 12.4. Complications of the Mainz pouch I procedure at the Department of Urology, University of Mainz, from 1983 to March 1992, in 314 patients

effectively treated by V-plasty of the efferent segment (Fig. 12.6a–c).

Stones have most commonly been found attached to staples (Figs 12.7 and 12.8). Using the appendix as a continence mechanism obviates this problem. After having created mesenteric windows and incising the taenia libera of the colon (Fig. 12.9), the appendix is embedded (Figs 12.10 and 12.11). This method of creating a continent outlet is preferred and used by the authors whenever possible. If the appendix is structurally altered and unusable, newer continence mechanisms such as a seromuscular tube[21] (Figs 12.12–12.14) or a tapered segment of ileum embedded in a taenia of the colon[22] are used (Figs 12.15–12.17).

To avoid diarrhoea or frequent bowel movements in patients with myelomeningocoele who undergo a Mainz pouch I continent urinary diversion, the ileocaecal valve is reconstructed (Figs 12.18–12.23).[23]

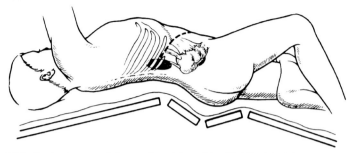

Figure 12.2. Optimal approach for pouch revision: right-sided flank incision.

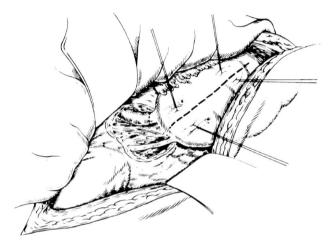

Figure 12.3. Flank incision leads directly to the site of ureterointestinal implantation. The pouch is opened parallel to the ureteral anastomosis site (dotted line).

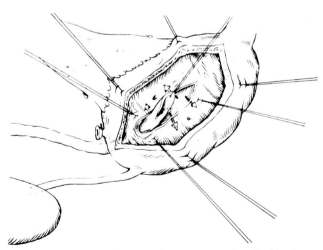

Figure 12.4. Creation of a wide 'button-hole' to accommodate the dilated ureter comfortably. After incision of the pouch mucosa, a wide, but short, submucosal tunnel is prepared.

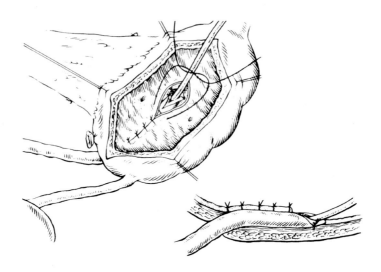

Figure 12.5. Two anchor sutures at 5 and 7 o'clock hold the ureter in position. The bowel mucosa is closed over the ureter with single-stitch sutures (catgut 5/0).

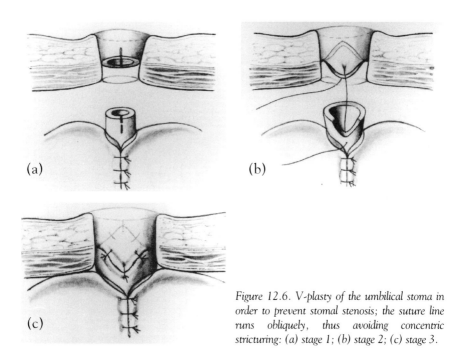

(a)

(b)

(c)

Figure 12.6. V-plasty of the umbilical stoma in order to prevent stomal stenosis; the suture line runs obliquely, thus avoiding concentric stricturing: (a) stage 1; (b) stage 2; (c) stage 3.

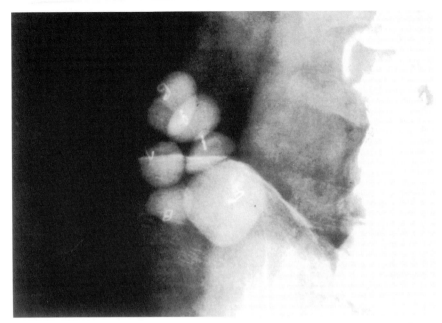

Figure 12.7. Plain X-ray film shows large stone development around staples in a Mainz pouch I.

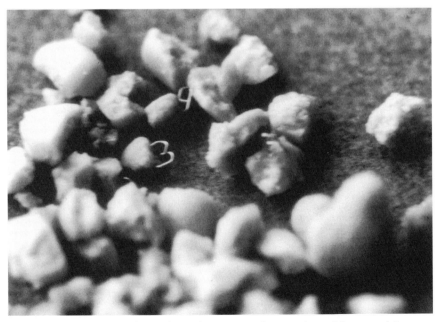

Figure 12.8. Stones attached to staples used to create an ileum nipple in a Mainz pouch I.

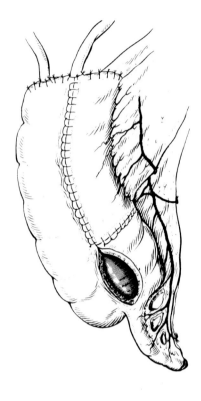

Figure 12.9. Excision of windows in the appendicular mesentery and incision of the taenia libera of the colon.

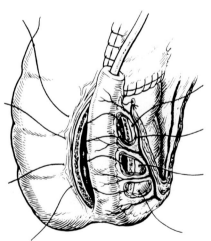

Figure 12.10. Placement of a 16 Fr silicone catheter through the appendix into the pouch. Seromuscular sutures (polyglycolic acid 4/0) are brought through the mesenteric windows in order to embed the appendix.

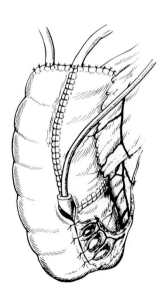

Figure 12.11. Closure of the seromuscular layer over the appendix with single-stitch sutures (polyglycolic acid 4/0).

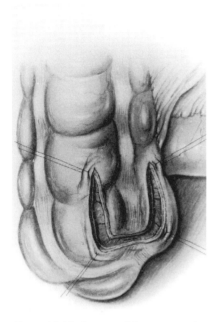

Figure 12.12. Incision of the seromuscular layer of the colon and careful separation of mucosa and seromuscularis laterally (1–2 mm).

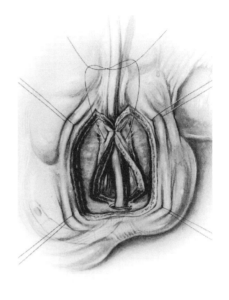

Figure 12.13. After a 5 mm incision of the mucosa at the proximal end of the seromuscular strip, a tube is formed over an 18 Fr silicone catheter with single-stitch sutures (polyglycolic acid 5/0).

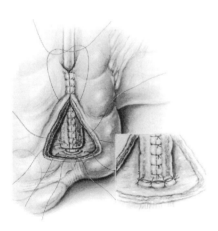

Figure 12.14. Anastomosis of the newly created tube with the mucosa of the colon (5/0 single-stitch sutures). Subsequently, the seromuscular layer is closed over the tube, thus submucosally embedding the continence mechanism.

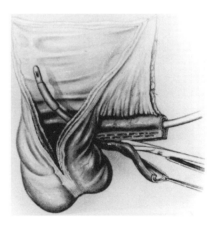

Figure 12.15. After insertion of a 14 Fr silicone catheter, the ileum is tapered and excess bowel discarded.

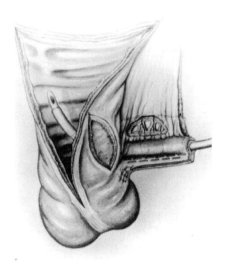

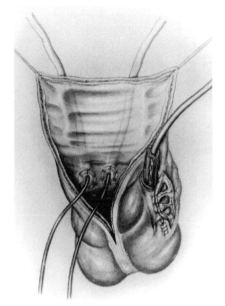

Figure 12.16. Oblique incision of the seromuscular layer between the taenia mesocolica and libera. Creation of mesenteric windows as described previously.

Figure 12.17. After placement of sutures through the mesenteric windows the seromuscular layer is closed using single-stitch sutures, thus embedding the tapered ileal segment.

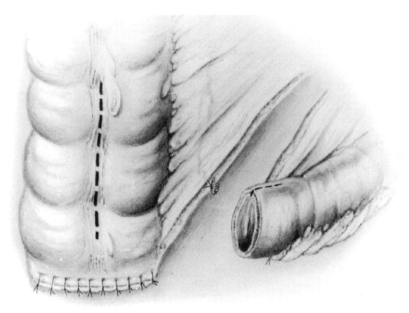

Figure 12.18. Terminal incision of the seromuscular layer of ascending colon over 6–7 cm and antimesenteric incision of terminal ileum. Incision of colonic mucosa over 2 cm (not shown).

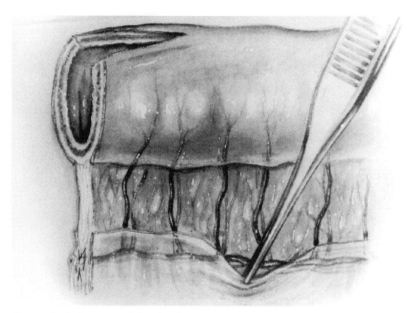

Figure 12.19. Mesentery defatted and serosa removed.

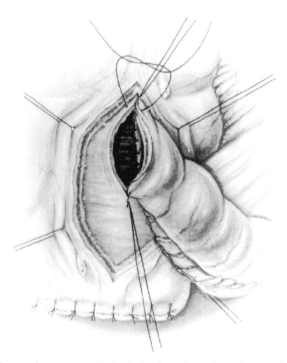

Figure 12.20. Ileocaecal anastomosis (5/0 polyglycolic acid, single-stitch sutures).

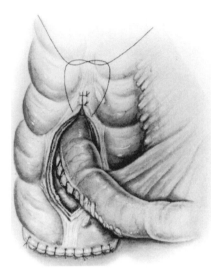

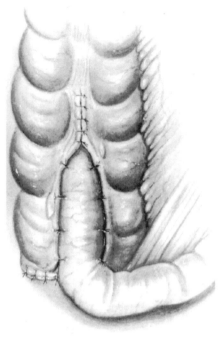

Figures 12.21 and 12.22. After closure of the seromuscular layer to create a submucosal tunnel 4 cm in length (see Fig. 16.2a in this volume), lateral sutures attach the ileum to the ileocaecal region in order to avoid kinking and obstruction.

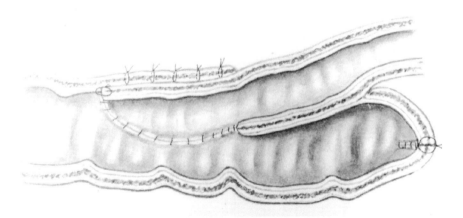

Figure 12.23. The lateral view depicts the ileum diving smoothly into the caecum.

For those patients with a competent anal sphincter and functionally damaged or morphologically absent urinary sphincter, the Mainz pouch II (sigma–rectum pouch) is a viable alternative (see also Chapter 17 of this volume). Preoperatively, anal sphincter competence is evaluated using a liquid enema. The patient has to be able to retain the saline enema for at least 3 h during the day while walking about and for many hours at night. In addition, a rectodynamic evaluation should give positive results[24]. Previous or planned radiotherapy is a contraindication for the Mainz pouch II procedure, as are pathological conditions of the sigmoid colon.

Since November 1990, 19 children have received a sigma–rectum pouch at the authors' institution. In these 19 children, three uretero-neoimplantation procedures were necessary in two children during two sessions. One child had an ileus 5 months after urinary diversion, which was revised by surgery. The obstruction at the site of the ureterointestinal anastomosis was caused by the use of slowly resorbable suture material. For this reason the authors now recommend the use of chromic catgut for ureteral implantation. The Mainz pouch II procedure is also indicated to correct failed ureterosigmoidostomy. For conversion surgery, a pre-existing antireflux colonic conduit can be incorporated into the sigma–rectum pouch, obviating the need for a new ureteral implantation procedure. Fixation of the pouch to the promontory or the psoas muscle prevents excess mobility, which might cause ureteral kinking and subsequent obstruction.

Types of urinary diversion and choice of intestinal segment

The need to convert incontinent forms of urinary diversion into continent types is occurring with increasing frequency. A total of 33 conversion procedures have been performed in young adults at the authors' institution (Fig. 12.24).[25] If, as mentioned above, a sigma–rectum pouch is not indicated because of anal sphincter incompetence, an antireflux colonic conduit (Figs 12.25–12.27) can also be incorporated into a Mainz pouch I continent reservoir (continent

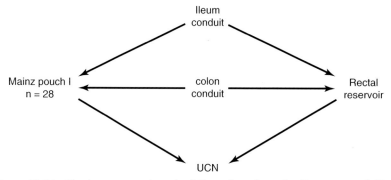

Figure 12.24. Continent conversions (n=33) performed at the Department of Urology, University of Mainz: UCN, ureterocutaneostomy. Data from ref. 25.

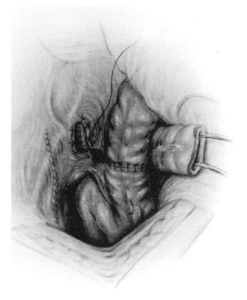

Figure 12.25. Correct positioning of colon conduit: after open transcolic ureteral implantation the cranial portion of the conduit is placed in the retroperitoneum.

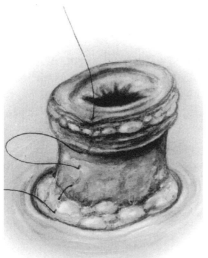

Figure 12.26. Stoma creation: suture grips the seromuscular layer and then the mucosa. Intracutaneous sutures preclude urinary fistulas.

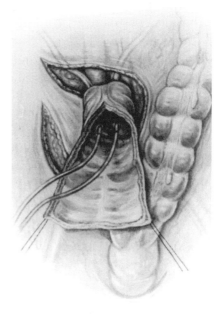

Figure 12.27. Antimesenteric opening of colonic conduit. Ureters stented.

conversion). Figures 12.28 and 12.29 illustrate how this can easily be achieved without the need for repeated ureteral implantation. Equally, the colonic conduit can be incorporated into a Mainz pouch II (Fig. 12.30a, b)

The choice of intestinal segment for urinary diversion is fraught with difficulty. Virtually every segment of the intestinal tract has been used in undiversion surgery and all have their specific advantages and disadvantages. Novel concepts such as incorporation of an isolated gastric segment have produced significant complications, as increasing experience and follow-up is showing.[26] Haematuria, alkalosis, dysuria and peptic ulcers in a 'dry' bladder have dampened most of the initial enthusiasm associated with the use of gastric segments.[27] Cases of perforation of the gastric segment of an augmented bladder secondary to peptic ulcer have even been reported.[28] The indications remaining are cloacal exstrophies and patients demonstrating compromised renal function.[29,30]

The ileum has certainly gained widespread popularity for the construction of continent reservoirs but here also long-term follow-up is demonstrating a significantly increased rate of complications at the site of ureterointestinal anastomosis. Antireflux ureteral implantation into an isolated segment of large bowel, which can also be used for augmentation, is technically simpler and reliably prevents reflux.

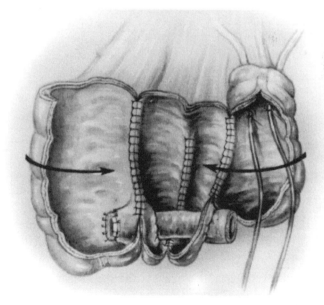

Figure 12.28. Side-to-side anastomosis of split colonic conduit to ileocaecal reservoir (Mainz pouch I).

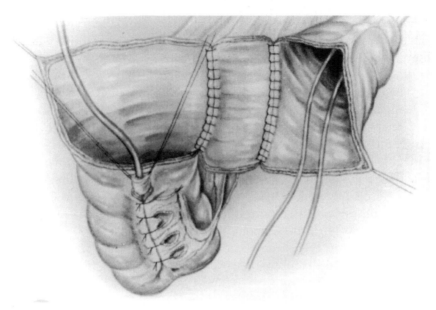

Figure 12.29. As Fig. 12.28 except that the appendix has been used as a continence mechanism, thus saving one loop of ileum.

(a) (b)

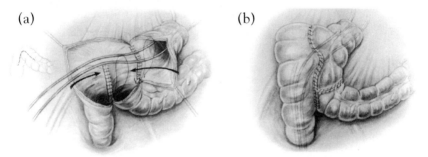

Figure 12.30. Side-to-side anastomosis of split colonic conduit to sigma–rectum pouch (Mainz pouch II): (a) stage 1; (b) stage 2.

When intermediary diversion or incontinent diversion has to be performed in order to stabilize or improve renal function, the colonic conduit should be preferred. The authors' series demonstrated that the condition of the upper urinary tract at the time of incontinent diversion is of the utmost importance and is a significant factor in predicting the outcome. From 1967 to 1983 the authors constructed a sigma conduit in 94 children with a mean age of 7.2 years at the time of operation. Of 124 preoperatively dilated renal units, 94 showed a decrease in dilatation postoperatively, whereas in ten units dilatation increased. Of 49 renal units that had pyelonephritic changes preoperatively, nine showed further changes during follow-up. In an additional two renal units, pyelonephritic changes were noted during the follow-up even though these changes were not present preoperatively. In the authors' opinion, dilated ureters and ureters with a thick and hypertrophied wall are prone to stricture at the implantation site and the risk of postoperative dilatation is severely increased. Intermediate diversion should therefore be performed at an early stage of disease and should not be considered as the ultimate solution.

Using the ileocaecal segment for urinary diversion affords the opportunity to construct a large-capacity low-pressure reservoir using a very small length of bowel. Ureteral implantation is easily accomplished in an antireflux manner using a simple and reproducible technique. Moreover, a wide variety of continence mechanisms may be used. Any supposed disadvantage attendant on resection of the ileocaecal valve can be obviated by reconstructing the valve surgically (see above).

Metabolic and neoplastic changes after urinary diversion

With regard to the metabolic consequences of urinary diversion, the possibility of vitamin deficiency and metabolic acidosis is the most pertinent issue. The authors have monitored the vitamin B_{12} level in 161 patients with a continent Mainz pouch I reservoir over a period of 6 years, and noted that it was markedly reduced when compared with an age-matched control group; the B_{12} level was, however, still within the normal range (Fig. 12.31). Similar results have been reported by other authors.[31] In a retrospective analysis of 130 patients after urinary diversion, Jahnson even found 11 patients with a vitamin B_{12} deficiency; however, all 11 patients had been irradiated preoperatively.[32] Routine evaluation of vitamin B_{12} serum levels should be carried out at follow-up. For such purposes B_{12} detection using the urinary methylmalonic acid test appears to be superior to serum B_{12} radioimmunoassays.[33,34]

More than 197 reports of neoplastic change occurring after ureterosigmoidostomy have been published to date. However, secondary tumours are also found in other types of urinary diversion; 32 cases have been reported so far in ileal conduits, colonic conduits and ileo- and colocystoplasties. In the authors' opinion, the close contact of urothelial epithelium and bowel mucosa is the most likely mechanism involved in secondary malignancy development. Consequently, the same risk of secondary malignancy should exist in every form of urinary diversion and, equally, in patients who have undergone bladder augmentation. Owing to the stasis of urine in continent reservoirs and augmented bladders, the risk of malignant transformation may be higher in these cases. Of the 17 secondary malignancies that were found in patients with

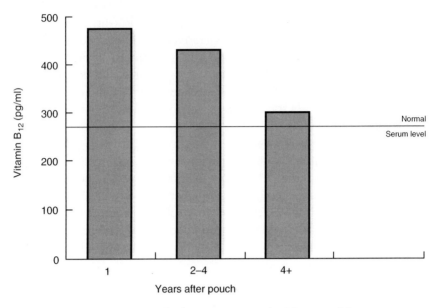

Figure 12.31. Vitamin B$_{12}$ serum levels in 161 patients after Mainz pouch I continent urinary diversion.

bladder augmentation, 11 occurred in ileocystoplasties and six in colocystoplasties, indicating that no difference exists in this respect between ileum and colon. Recent research has suggested that metaplasia may also follow gastrocystoplasty.[35]

The latent period for detection in humans is, on average, 18 years.[36] Because ureterosigmoidostomy has been used very much longer than any other form of urinary diversion, it has the highest reported incidence of secondary malignancies. Nevertheless, the ureterointestinal anastomosis must be examined regularly; those reservoirs are to be preferred, therefore, that allow easy access for such investigations. Specially developed instruments facilitate this examination by providing variable degrees of magnification.

If malignancy is suspected during optical evaluation of the ureteral implantation site, a biopsy can easily be performed. In the case of grade 3 dysplasia, conversion to another form of continent urinary diversion is possible. Continent urinary diversion has been shown to be advantageous in such cases as the patient is not confronted with an incontinent stoma that would cause additional dismay.[37]

Acidosis as a result of urinary diversion must be corrected if the base excess drops below –2.5. This is prevention and not treatment. The situation is comparable to that of a diabetic patient; no one would wait until a diabetic coma develops until insulin is administered, but inspection of the follow-up programmes of many institutions indicates that this is exactly what is being done with regard to urinary diversion. Acidosis must be corrected at an early stage by administration of alkalinizing drugs before dangerous levels are reached and most certainly before hyperchloraemia develops.

What will the future bring?

An increasing number of publications dealing with bladder augmentation using dilated ureteral tissue have been published recently.[38-41] Interestingly, none of these papers has cited the author who first described ureterocystoplasty — Herbert Eckstein — who first used a dilated ureter for augmentation and reported this technique in 1973.[42] The patient subsequently underwent renal transplantation, demonstrated a functionally normal bladder after augmentation and was able to void through the urethra. The early results of ureterocystoplasty compare favourably with those of enterocystoplasty in selected cases, but further experience and follow-up are certainly required.

Similar advances have been made in constructing a continent vesicostomy (Figs 12.32–12.38). As an alternative to the Mitrofanoff principle,[43] which has many disadvantages,[44-46] the use of a submucosally embedded bladder flap is a promising novel development.[25,47]

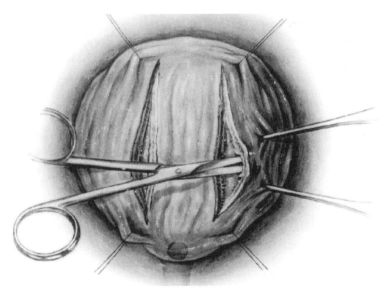

Figure 12.32. Preparation of a 3 × 8 cm seromuscular 'Boari' flap and careful lateral mobilization of mucosa.

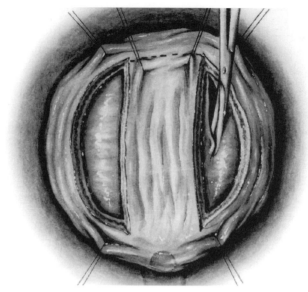

Figure 12.33. Opening the bladder lateral to the flap.

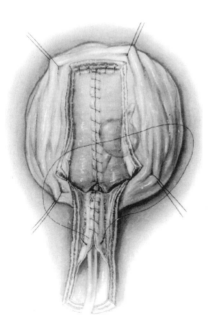

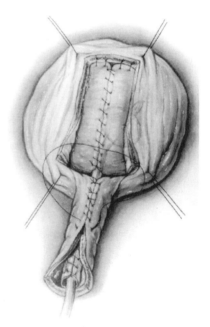

Figure 12.34. Closure of bladder mucosa using a running suture and adaptation of mucosa over a 18 Fr silicone catheter.

Figure 12.35. Closure of seromuscular layer over tube.

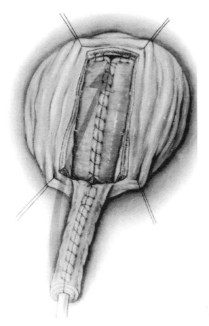

Figure 12.36. Newly created tube is subsequently laid back into submucosal bed.

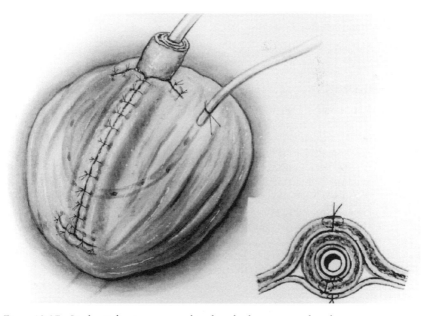

Figure 12.37. Single-stitch sutures are used to close the detrusor over the tube.

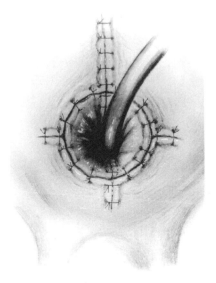

Figure 12.38. Creation of pseudoumbilical stoma.

In conclusion, it must be realized that construction of a worthy alternative to the natural bladder is still a distant goal. Nevertheless, substantial progress has been made. All reconstructive surgery of the lower urinary tract is, by nature, burdened with specific problems. However, by carefully considering the advantages and disadvantages of each technique, the procedure that is most beneficial for the individual patient can be pinpointed.

References

1. Light J K, Scott F B. The artificial urinary sphincter in children. Br J Urol 1984; 56: 54–75
2. Gonzalez R, Sheldon C A. Artificial sphincters in children with neurogenic bladders: long-term results. J Urol 1982; 128: 1270–1272
3. Aprikian A, Berardinucci G, Pike J, Kiruluta G. Experience with the AS-800 artificial urinary sphincter in myelodysplastic children. Can J Surg 1992; 35: 396–400
4. Bosco P J, Bauer S B, Colodny A H et al. The long-term results of artificial sphincters in children. J Urol 1991; 146: 396–399
5. Grein U, Schreiter F. Le sphincter artificiel chez l'enfant. J Urol (Paris) 1990; 2: 93–96
6. Barrett D M, Parulkar B G. The artificial sphincter (AS-800). Experience in children and young adults. Urol Clin North Am 1989; 16: 1–32
7. Nurse D E, Mundy A R. One hundred artificial sphincters. Br J Urol 1988; 61: 318–325
8. Reinberg Y, Manviel J C, Gonzalez R. Silicone shedding from artificial urinary sphincter in children. J Urol 1993; 150: 694–696

9. Jones J A, Mitchell M E, Rink R C. Improved results using a modification of the Young–Dees–Leadbetter bladder neck repair. Br J Urol 1993; 71: 555–561

10. Kramer S A, Kelalis P P. Assessment of urinary continence in epispadias: review of 94 patients. J Urol 1982; 128: 290–293

11. Hollowell J G, Ransley P G. Surgical management of incontinence in bladder exstrophy. Br J Urol 1991; 61: 534

12. Gearhart J P, Jeffs R D. Augmentation cystoplasty in failed exstrophy reconstruction. J Urol 1988; 139: 790–793

13. Gearhart J P, Williams K A, Jeffs R D. Intraoperative urethral pressure profilometry as an adjunct to bladder neck reconstruction. J Urol 1986; 136: 1055–1056

14. Hollowell J G, Hill P D, Duffy P G, Ransley P G. Bladder function and dysfunction in exstrophy and epispadias. Lancet 1991; 338: 926–928

15. Hollowell J G, Hill P D, Duffy P G, Ransley P G. Lower urinary tract function after exstrophy closure. Pediatr Nephrol 1992; 6: 428–432

16. Hollowell J G, Hill P D, Duffy P G, Ransley P G. Evaluation and treatment of incontinence after bladder neck reconstruction in exstrophy and epispadias. Br J Urol 1993; 71: 743–749

17. Kazachkov S A, Derzhavin V M, Bannikov V M, Berulava Z O. [The urodynamics of the lower urinary tract after reconstructive operations in bladder exstrophy.] Urol Nefrol (Mosk) 1990; 7–10

18. McGuire E J, Bennett C I, Konnak I A. Experience with pubovaginal slings for urinary incontinence at the University of Michigan. J Urol 1987; 138: 525–526

19. Raz S, Siegel A L, Short J L, Snyder J A. Vaginal wall sling. J Urol 1989; 141: 43–46

20. Decter R M. Use of the fascial sling for neurogenic incontinence: lessons learned. J Urol 1993; 150: 683–686

21. Lampel A, Hohenfellner M, Schultz-Lampel D et al. Submuköser Seromuskularis-Conduit: Eine neue Technik des kontinenten Stomas beim Mainz-Pouch. Aktuel Urol 1993; 24: I–VIII

22. Managadze L, Tschigogidze T. Tiflis-Pouch. Aktuel Urol 1993; 24: I–VI

23. Fisch M, Wammack R, Spies F et al. Ileocecal valve reconstruction during continent urinary diversion. J Urol 1994; 151: 861–865

24. Wammack R, Fisch M, Müller S C, Hohenfellner R. The rectodynamic evaluation. Assessment of anal continence in urology. Scand J Urol Nephrol 1992; 142 (Suppl 158)

25. Wammack R, Fisch M, Hohenfellner R. Conversion and undiversion surgery. Urologia 1993; 60: 127–134

26. Sumfest J M, Mitchell M E. Gastrocystoplasty in children. Eur Urol 1994; 25: 89–93

27. Nguyen D H, Bain M A, Salmonson K L et al. The syndrome of dysuria and hematuria in pediatric urinary reconstruction with stomach. J Urol 1993; 150: 707–709

28. Reinberg Y, Manivel J C, Froemming C, Gonzales R. Performation of the gastric segment of an augmented bladder secondary to peptic ulcer disease. J Urol 1992; 148: 369–371

29. Burns M W, Watkins S L, Mitchell M E, Tapper D. Treatment of bladder dysfunction in children with end-stage renal disease. J Pediatr Surg 1992; 27: 170–174

30. Steffens J, Sumfest J M. Gastrocystoplasty in children: a method limited to specific cases. Eur Urol 1994; 26: 270

31. Steiner M S, Mortin R A, Marshall F F. Vitamin B12 deficiency in patients with ileocolic neobladders. J Urol 1993; 149: 255–257

32. Jahnson S, Pedersen J. Cystectomy and urinary diversion during twenty years — complications and metabolic implications. Eur Urol 1993; 24: 343–349

33. Norman E J, Morrison J A. Screening elder populations for cobalamin (vitamin B12) deficiency using the urinary methylmalonic acid assay by gas chromatography mass spectometry. Am J Med 1993; 94: 589–595

34. Norman E J. Detection of cobalamin deficiency using the urinary methylmalonic acid test by gas chromatography mass spectrometry. J Clin Pathol 1993; 46: 382

35. Klee L W, Hoover D M, Mitchell M E, Rink R C. Long term effects of gastrocystoplasty in rats. J Urol 1990; 144: 1283–1287

36. Filmer B, Spencer J R. Malignancies in bladder augmentations and intestinal conduits. J Urol 1990; 143: 671

37. Woodhouse C R J. Long-term peadiatric urology. Oxford: Blackwell Scientific Publications, 1991: 80–96

38. Churchill B M, Aliabadi H, Landau E H et al. Ureteral bladder augmentation. J Urol 1993; 150: 716–720

39. Wolf J S Jr, Turzan C W. Augmentation ureterocystoplasty, J Urol 1993; 149: 1095–1098

40. Bellinger M F. Ureterocystoplasty: a unique method for vesical augmentation in children. J Urol 1993; 149: 811–813

41. Hitchcock R J I, Duffy P G, Malone P S. Ureterocystoplasty: the 'bladder' augmentation of choice. Br J Urol 1994; 73: 575–579

42. Eckstein H B, Martin M R R. Uretero-Cystoplastik. Aktuel Urol 1973; 4: 255–257

43. Mitrofanoff P. Cystostomie continente transappendiculaire dans le traitement des vessies neurologiques. Chir Pediatr 1980; 21: 297

44. Montfort G, Guys J M, Lacombe G M. Appendicovesicostomy: an alternative urinary diversion in the child. Eur Urol 1984; 10: 361

45. Duckett J W, Snyder H M III. Continent urinary diversion: variations of the Mitrofanoff principle. J Urol 1986; 136: 58

46. Woodhouse C R J, Malone P R, Cumming J, Reilly T M. The Mitrofanoff principle for continent urinary diversion. Br J Urol 1989; 63: 53

47. Hohenfellner R. Ausgewählte urologische OP-Techniken. Stuttgart: Thieme; 1994: 227

13

Mitrofanoff procedure in the absence of appendix: alternatives for urinary continence in complicated paediatric reconstructions

A. B. Retik   R. N. Schlussel
M. C. Carr   C. A. Peters   J. Mandell
S. B. Bauer   A. Atala   A. H. Colodny

Introduction

Few procedures can be as satisfying to paediatric patients, their parents, paediatricians and urologists, as one that converts the patient from incontinence to a dry state. A multitude of procedures have been devised to achieve such a goal. These innovations, in combination with the demonstration of the safety and efficacy of clean intermittent catheterization, have greatly improved continence rates in previously incontinent children. For an incontinent procedure to be accepted it should be technically easy to perform, have few complications, consistently achieve the desired goal of continence and result in reliable catheterization.

The Mitrofanoff procedure fulfils these criteria and therefore became quite popular in the surgical community.[1-6] In his original paper, Mitrofanoff[7] proposed isolating the appendix on its blood supply. The appendix tip is tunnelled into the bladder in a submucosal fashion, with the appendiceal base brought to the abdominal wall as a stoma for catheterization. Continence is achieved by means of the flap valve mechanism: the hydrostatic pressure of the full bladder compresses the submucosal appendix and prevents leakage of urine.

Although this is an effective procedure, many patients who present for reconstruction lack an appendix. An alternative solution is to tunnel other organs similarly into the urinary reservoir and then to use these organs as catheterizable conduits. In this chapter, the authors describe their experience in employing organs other than the appendix, using the Mitrofanoff principle to achieve urinary continence.

Patient data

From the years 1986 to 1993, continent diversions using the Mitrofanoff principle were carried out in 19 (12 male and seven female) patients. The patients' ages ranged from 3 years and 7 months to 20 years, with an average of 13 years. The indications for the procedure were exstrophy of the bladder (seven patients), spinal dysraphism (six patients), cystectomy for tumour (three patients) and miscellaneous conditions (three patients). The urinary reservoirs were three bladders, six augmented bladders (three sigmoid, two gastric, one ileal), five ileocaecal pouches, two sigmoid pouches, two gastric–transverse colon composites, and one ileal–sigmoid composite. The catheterizable conduits were fashioned from 14 ureters, four tapered ileum and one gastric tube.

Follow-up ranged from 4 months to 8 years, with an average follow-up of 30 months.

Results and complications

Total continence was achieved in 18 of the 19 patients. One patient was occasionally incontinent when catheterization was delayed for more than 4 h. There were six complications related to the catheterizable conduit: these comprised two stomal stenoses, one enteric fistula and one vesicourethral fistula and, in two patients, inability to catheterize themselves.

Discussion

A variety of surgical techniques have evolved which have reversed urinary incontinence in almost all clinical situations. The authors' preference is to work with the native bladder and urethra and to avoid diversion to achieve continence; in most instances this is possible. However, in some circumstances (such as wheelchair-bound patients unable to pass a catheter, and those who have undergone radiation therapy and/or cystectomy) a continent diversion is necessary in order for the patient to become dry. The Mitrofanoff procedure is one such diversion. As outlined above, in Mitrofanoff's original paper the procedure was described as harvesting the appendix on its blood supply, then tunnelling the tip submucosally into the bladder; the appendix base is then brought to the skin as a catheterizable stoma. In order to make a short appendix of adequate length, the base of the caecum can be incorporated in continuity with the appendix by use of a stapling device.[8] The appendix has proved to be a reliable efferent limb both for achieving continence and allowing patients to catheterize.

However, in many cases the appendix is either unavailable or unsuitable for reconstruction. Despite this inability to use the appendix, the Mitrofanoff principle, namely continence by means of the flap valve mechanisms, can still be employed. Other viscous, pliable organs can be placed in a submucosal tunnel and brought to the skin for catheterization. Several papers either have described modifications of the Mitrofanoff procedure[9–11] or have explored the use of other tubes including the vas deferens,[4] bladder tubes[12] and fallopian tubes.[13] When the appendix has been unavailable, the present authors have used the ureter, ileum or stomach.

Frequently, the ureter is the most straightforward option because it is already in position in the urinary reservoir in an antireflux fashion. The ureter is divided at a point that will allow the distal portion enough length to reach the abdominal wall and the proximal portion enough length to perform a transureteroureterostomy (TUU). As in other ureteral procedures, the ureter should be mobilized with the maximum amount of periureteral tissue to preserve ureteral blood supply and to prevent complications of ischaemia. Neither the proximal nor distal segments of the ureter should be angulated and the TUU should be a spatulated, stented anastomosis. Adhering to these principles enables any complications from the TUU or the distal ureter to be avoided. In one patient in the authors' series, a refluxing ureter was reimplanted and its proximal portion was brought to the skin. In cases as these, when operating on both ends of the ureter, the reimplantation should be performed by means of the Lich–Gregoir technique in order to avoid compromising the ureteral blood supply.

When the ileum is employed, a section is isolated on its mesentery and bowel continuity is re-established. The length of ileum harvested is dependent on the position of the reservoir and the patient's body habitus. The isolated ileum is narrowed on its antimesenteric side to limit wandering or kinking of the catheter; this narrowing can be done rapidly with a stapling device (Fig. 13.1). Stones should not form on these staples, as they will not be exposed to urine. The length of the ileum should be planned carefully; if the segment is too long, efforts to shorten the ileal segment may involve compromising its main blood supply. A narrowed ileum can be implanted into the urinary reservoir. Adequate flaps of the seromuscular layer or the taenia coli of the reservoir should be made so that the closure over the larger ileum can be made without tension. This technique can also be used to convert an ileal conduit to a catheterizable conduit.[14]

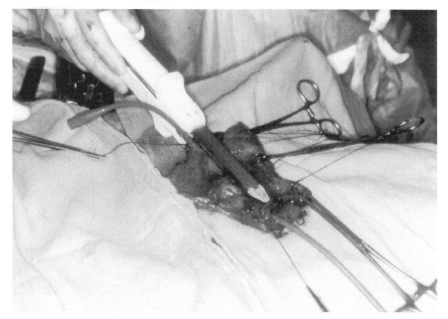

Figure 13.1. The isolated ileum is tapered on its antimesenteric border over a 12 Fr catheter with the use of a gastrointestinal stapling device.

A stomach tube is one more option to use as a catheterizable stoma. The blood supply for this tube is based on the gastroepiploic artery, as in a gastrocystoplasty. This tube can be similarly implanted into any urinary reservoir, and then brought to the abdominal wall for catheterization (Fig. 13.2). There have been other isolated reports of gastric tubes used for catheterization with similar success.[1,15]

In order for catheterization to proceed easily, the efferent limb must be straight. Excess length of this limb can lead to looping or kinking of the catheter. The authors have found that suturing the limb, the reservoir or both to the anterior abdominal wall will ensure a consistently straight path for the catheter to traverse. The temptation to close the abdomen if there is any difficulty with the catheterization should be resisted strenuously, because hopes that these difficulties will resolve spontaneously postoperatively are rarely fulfilled.

The authors have not encountered any complications related to the efferent limb in their last seven patients. This is attributable in part to the advantage of experience, as well at to the use of a V flap of skin in constructing the stoma. To create such a V flap, a triangle of skin is marked with the tip abutting the circular skin defect created for the stoma. The triangular skin is undermined, and the tip of the flap is sutured to the apex of a spatulation made in the efferent limb. This flap

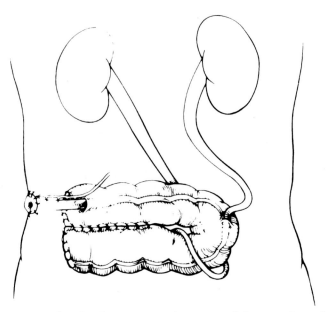

Figure 13.2. A gastric tube is based on a gastroepiploic artery pedicle; one end is implanted into the colonic reservoir and the other end is brought to the abdominal wall for catheterization.

has a dual purpose: interposition of the broad flap base into the circumference of the efferent limb widens the stoma circumference and thereby reduces the risk of a stomal stenosis; in addition, the flap enables the stoma to be partially recessed for an improved cosmetic appearance.

The authors prefer to use the umbilicus as the stoma site, when possible, as it affords easy access for catheterization and is less noticeable than other sites on the abdominal wall.

Correct patient selection is of great importance in any procedure that will require future catheterization. In almost all instances, the authors reserve such a continence procedure for the child who is old enough to demonstrate both the ability and the motivation to catheterize on a regular basis; this age usually corresponds to the time of puberty. The creation of a continent diversion that requires catheterization in a patient who cannot or will not do so can result in a catastrophe.

In conclusion, the authors' experience has shown that the absence of an appendix does not preclude the use of the Mitrofanoff principle. Ureter, ileum and stomach can be readily implanted in the bladder or urinary pouch so that urine filling the pouch will cause coaptation of the efferent limbs and prevent leakage. Familiarity with these alternatives expands the armamentarium of the reconstructive surgeon. These efferent limbs can result in satisfactory rates of continence and reliable catheterization and are effective alternatives to the appendix in urinary continence procedures.

References

1. Borzi P A, Bruce J, Gough D C. Continent cutaneous diversions in children: experience with the Mitrofanoff procedure. Br J Urol 1992; 70: 669–673
2. Elder J S. Continent appendicocolostomy: a variation of the Mitrofanoff principle in pediatric urinary tract reconstruction. J Urol 1992; 148: 117–119
3. Cendron M, Gearhart J P. The Mitrofanoff principle. Technique and application in continent urinary diversion. Urol Clin North Am 1991; 18: 615–621
4. Dykes E H, Duffy P G, Ransley P G. The use of the Mitrofanoff principle in achieving clean intermittent catheterisation and urinary continence in children. J Pediatr Surg 1991; 26: 535–538
5. Hensle T W, Connor J P, Burbige K A. Continent urinary diversion in childhood. J Urol 1990; 143: 981–983
6. Weingarten J L, Cromie W J. The Mitrofanoff principle: an alternative form of continent urinary diversion. J Urol 1988; 140: 1529–1531
7. Mitrofanoff P. Cystostomie continente trans-appendiculaire dans le traitement des vessies neurologiques. Chir Pediatr 1980; 21: 297
8. Cromie W J, Barada J H, Weingarten J L. Cecal tubularization: lengthening technique for creation of catheterizable conduit. Urology 1991; 37: 41–42
9. Keetch D W, Basler J W, Kavoussi L R, Catalona W J. Modification of the Mitrofanoff principle for continent urinary diversion. Urology 1993; 41: 507–510
10. Duckett J W, Lotfi A H. Appendicovesicostomy (and variations) in bladder reconstruction. J Urol 1993; 149: 567–569
11. Duckett J W, Snyder H M III. The Mitrofanoff principle in continent urinary reservoirs. Semin Urol 1987; 5: 55–62
12. Klabuer G T, Cendron M. Continent vesicostomy using a catheterizable posterior bladder tube: modification of the Mitrofanoff principle. J Pediatr Surg 1994; 29: 71–73
13. Woodhouse C R, Malone P R, Cumming J, Reilly T M. The Mitrofanoff principle for continent urinary diversion. Br J Urol 1989; 63: 53–57
14. Adams M C, Bihrle R, Foster R S, Brito C G. Conversion of an ileal conduit to a continent catheterizable stoma. J Urol 1992; 147: 126–128
15. Borzi P, Gauch D C. Pedicled gastric tube as a catheterising conduit. Eur Urol 1993; 24: 103–105

14

Urinary diversion and fertility in bladder exstrophy patients

R. Stein   M. Fisch   M. Stöckle
R. Hohenfellner

Introduction

Bladder exstrophy is a rare but devasting condition with an incidence of 1:33 000 newborns; the male-to-female ratio is 1.5:1.[1] Incontinent epispadias is even less common (1:42 000). As a result of modern operative techniques and highly improved postoperative medical care, these children today have a normal life expectancy.[2,3]

The two pillars of treatment of bladder exstrophy are achievement of complete urinary continence and reconstruction of the external — and in females additionally the internal — genitalia. Numerous methods of treatment have been reported; however, the optimal surgical procedure still remains a matter of debate.[3-10] Primary bladder closure with or without osteotomy followed later by bladder neck reconstruction and bilateral ureteroneocystostomy still represents the most common operative procedure for correction of these anomalies.[5] Continence varies from institution to institution (from 32% to over 80%),[4,6] with a rate of reoperations of up to 75% and deterioration of the urinary upper tract in 24%.[7] During the last few years the continence rate has improved in the hands of experienced surgeons and carefully selected patients. The definition of continence includes patients who are able to empty their bladder only by clean intermittent catheterization (CIC), in male patients at the risk of recurrent epididymitis and/or urethral strictures. Incontinence, on the other hand, is associated with many psychosocial problems for children and parents. The optimal approach should achieve continence during both the day and the night before children reach school age.

An alternative has been offered by ureterosigmoidostomy, which has been the urinary diversion technique of choice for more than 20 years and results in a continence rate of 93%.[9] Recently, the procedure has been modified to include a sigma rectum pouch (Mainz pouch II) created by antimesenteric opening of the rectosigmoid and side-to-side anastomosis, thus offering the advantage of a low-pressure reservoir.[11] In patients with an insufficient anal sphincter mechanism or short ureters with a thick wall, the authors construct an ileocaecal pouch with a continent umbilical stoma (Mainz pouch I). An intermediate colon conduit with the option of conversion to continent urinary diversion is constructed in patients with a dilated upper tract; this provides the advantage of a low pressure system, leading to stabilization or recovery of renal function.[12]

There have been numerous reports on the techniques and success rates of genital reconstruction.[5] In women, reconstruction of the external genitalia is uncomplicated. Fertility is normal if the internal genitalia are intact; severe complications of pregnancy are not to be expected.[2,3,13] However, uterine prolapse has been reported, especially after an introitusplasty.[2,13,14] Much more likely to cause complications is the reconstruction of the external male genitalia, although the majority of the patients have reportedly been satisfied with the cosmetic results.[15] The effect of genital reconstruction on sexuality, and especially fertility, has been rather neglected in the literature, as a very low fertility rate of only 8–18% has been reported.[3,16] The latter factor represents a serious personal problem for the male patient.

The authors here report their experience in patients with bladder exstrophy or incontinent epispadias over a quarter of a century and discuss the operative opportunities and their risks with regard to renal function, sexuality and, last but not least, fertility.

Patients and methods

Since 1968, 20 patients with incontinent epispadias and 95 with bladder exstrophy have undergone surgery at the authors' institution. A total of 104 patients could be followed. One patient with serious family problems refused to participate: ten of the 115 patients were lost during follow-up, nine of whom had moved out of the country.

During the follow-up period two patients died, one of liver failure due to alcohol toxicity and one of signet ring cell carcinoma of the unclosed bladder. Mean follow-up since the first operative intervention was 16.7 years (0.2–35 years). In 34 patients, the follow-up period was more than 20 years. Regular follow-up examinations were performed in 82 patients. The follow-up data of the remaining 20 patients were obtained by questionnaire or by telephone. In all patients an ultrasound examination of the kidney and determination of the serum creatinine levels have been performed during the last 18 months, either at the authors' institution or by an external urologist or paediatrician.

Results

Ureterosigmoidostomy, as the primary standard procedure, was performed in 26 of the patients followed. At the time of operation only six were older than 1 year and three older than 6 years (7–21 years). Ureterosigmoidostomy was also done in nine additional patients after failure of the previous operation (in seven of these after primary bladder closure and/or bladder neck reconstruction). Of these 35 patients, 29 individuals (83%) still have this type of urinary diversion. Early postoperative complications were two cases of acute abdominal wall dehiscence and one of ileus. In ten out of 35 patients, patients stenosis of the ureter occurred; one of these patients previously had an ileal conduit and one a primary bladder closure; preoperatively, two already showed dilatation of the upper urinary tract. Ureters were reimplanted in six of the 35 patients. To preserve renal function, a conversion to colon conduit had to be performed in five patients, in one of whom the conversion took place after failure of the ureteral neoimplantation. Owing to incontinence in one girl, a conversion to an ileocaecal pouch was carried out. Nephrectomy was necessary in two patients. In one woman a partial nephrectomy was performed 20 years after ureterosigmoidostomy, because of stones and subsequent pyelonephritis.

Because of complications attributable to urinary diversion or unsatisfactory cosmetic results of the reconstruction of the external genitalia, 12 patients with ureterosigmoidostomy that had been performed in another hospital were referred to the authors' institution. This highly selected group had a high complication rate. Stenosis of the ureters necessitated conversion to a colon conduit in three and to a sigma–rectum pouch in one of the 12 patients (33%). In one female patient the colon conduit was later incorporated in a sigma–rectum pouch. Incontinence necessitated conversion to a Mainz pouch I in five patients.

At the time of writing, in 32 patients with ureterosigmoidostomy a follow-up has been possible. All have normal serum creatinine values and none showed upper tract dilatation on ultrasound examination. One male patient had pyelonephritis in 1993, five patients pass some drops of urine during the night (requiring only one incontinence pad), but this occurs mostly during illness. One patient is incontinent. Five patients require oral antiacidosis treatment for compensation of metabolic acidosis (sodium potassium citrate). Of the older patients, 14 undergo regular sigmoidoscopy without any pathological findings (Table 14.1).

A *Mainz pouch II* was constructed in 17 patients, in nine as the primary urinary diversion and after failure of bladder closure/bladder neck repair in three. The remaining five patients had experienced

Conversion		n = 38
(More than one conversion		n = 3)
Incontinent to continent (requested by the patient)		n = 12
Conduit to	Ureterosigmoidostomy/Mainz pouch II	n = 3
	Mainz pouch I	n = 4
TUUC† to	Mainz pouch I/Mainz pouch II	n = 5
Continent to continent (failure)		n = 15
Other rectal reservoirs to	Ureterosigmoidostomy/Mainz pouch II	n = 3
	Mainz pouch I	n = 3
Ureterosigmoidostomy to	Mainz pouch I	n = 8
	Mainz pouch II	n = 1
Continent to incontinent (failure)		n = 9
Other rectal reservoir to	Colon conduit	n = 1
Ureterosigmoidostomy to	Colon conduit	n = 8
Incontinent to incontinent (failure)		n = 2
Ileal conduit to	Colon conduit	n = 2

* Even if performed at a different hospital.
† TUUC, Transureterocureterocutaneostomy.

*Table 14.1. Conversion in all patients with follow-up**

incontinent urinary diversion (three), stenosis of the ureter after ureterosigmoidostomy (one) and failure of the Boyce Vest reconstruction (one); in the latter patient a primary bladder closure had failed previously.

Follow-up was possible in 16 of the 17 patients. A 7-year-old Arab boy who had had incontinent epispadias, and who was continent when he returned home 2 months after the operation, is lost to follow-up. Ureteral stenosis ocurred in three, necessitating reimplantation. One girl had an ileus 8 months after the reimplantation. An upper tract dilatation of one kidney was found in one female patient with two previous operations; however, there was no change compared with the degree of dilatation before the first intervention. None of the others showed any significant dilatation on ultrasound examination or i.v. pyelogram at the last check-up (Fig. 14.1). Only one 17-year-old girl has slight stress incontinence. Of the 16 patients, 10 required alkalizing agents.

A *modified Young–Dees procedure with Mainz pouch augmentation* was performed in eight boys and one girl. One boy is lost to follow-up. In one boy, reimplantation of both ureters was necessary 8 months after operation. Owing to obstruction in four and complete incontinence in one, a total of five patients require conversion to a Mainz pouch I with a continent stoma; the other three patients have a normal upper urinary tract. Two are completely continent, one with residual urine in the augmented bladder of about 40 ml. One girl who had had epispadias is partially incontinent day and night, but under biofeedback training the situation is tolerable for her and her parents.

A *Mainz pouch I* was constructed in 31 patients. All 30 living patients could be followed, 17 after failed primary bladder closure and/or bladder neck reconstruction. Because of the patient's wish for continence, or after failure of other types of urinary diversion, a Mainz pouch I was created in 13 patients, in four of whom a previously constructed conduit was integrated. Necrosis of the nipple occurred soon after the operation in one male patient; he needs an external collection device, but has no

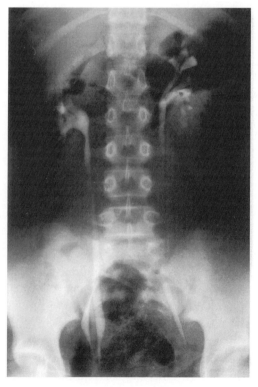

Figure 14.1. Pyelography in a 13-year-old girl with ureterocutaneostomy after failure of bladder closure; conversion to a sigma rectum pouch was performed at the age of 12 years (see Fig. 17.1, this volume).

problems with this solution and does not want a continent stoma. Two female patients underwent reimplantation of the ureter because of two stenoses at the implantation site; two stoma stenoses could be treated by simple incision; one traumatic pouch rupture (car accident) required surgical repair. One man in whom urinary tract reconstruction had failed previously (about five operations) showed dilation of the upper urinary tract postoperatively. No patient has shown deterioration of the upper urinary tract and all patients had normal serum creatinine values. In 97% of the patients there is complete continence by day and by night; eight patients require alkalizing agents for correction of the acid–base balance (Table 14.2).

A primary *intermediate colon conduit* was constructed in five children with a dilated upper urinary tract. The conduit was integrated into a Mainz pouch I in one girl when she was 11 years of age, and in another girl into a colon–rectum pouch when she was 5 years old; the latter girl needs pads. The remaining three patients with a primary colon conduit are still waiting for conversion to continent urinary diversion: two are too young at present and one man wishes to complete his education first. After failure of urinary tract reconstruction, a colon conduit was constructed in 12 patients with a dilated urinary upper tract, to preserve renal function. One stoma stenosis required an open revision and two ureteral stenoses were followed by reimplantation in one patient and a nephrectomy in the other. In three of the 12 patients a conversion is planned; nine patients with a secondary colon conduit are satisfied with their situation and do not want a continent urinary diversion. All patients except one boy now have a normal upper urinary tract, confirmed by ultrasound examination, normal creatinine values and no need for correction of the acid–base balance.

Procedure	Continence (no. of patients)	(%)
Rectal reservoirs (ureterosigmoidostomy/Mainz pouch II)	47/50	94
Mainz pouch I	29/30	97
Modified Young–Dees (Mainz pouch augmentation)	2/3	67
Sling plasty	1/2	50

Table 14.2. Current continence rates in patients undergoing urinary diversion for bladder exstrophy

None of 102 living patients with follow-up has renal insufficiency and none developed bowel neoplasia.

Sexuality and fertility

Of the adult patients followed up, 34 are married or have a steady partner. Reconstruction of the external genitalia was performed in 25 of 37 girls at an average age of 12.2 years (2.5–27 years). Reconstructive surgery included approximation of the divergent mons pubis and bifid clitoris, and reconstruction of the labia minora, whenever possible, in 25 patients. Vaginal cut-back or vaginoplasty was performed in 23 patients; in 13 instances this was associated with reconstruction of the external genitalia. Prolapse occurred several months later in four patients, three of whom subsequently underwent fixation of the uterus; a pessary was recommended by the gynaecologist to the other patient. As a result of this experience, the authors undertook fixation of the uterus in the same session as vaginal cut-back in 10 further cases: antefixation of the uterus was carried out in 11 women (Fig. 14.2) and the 'Kocher' procedure[17] in two. The average age at operation was 19 years (13–27 years).

Two adult patients with incontinent epispadias and sling plasty have not yet undergone genital reconstruction, and it is planned for the future in five young girls with epispadias.

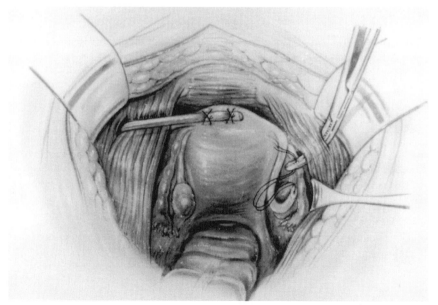

Figure 14.2. Antefixation of the uterus: together with the suture the ligamentum rotundum is pulled through from the internal to the external side of the rectus muscle and fixed at the uterus.

Of 17 adult females with reconstruction of the external genitalia, 16 are satisfied with the cosmetic results achieved by correction of the external genitalia and vaginal cut-back. No recurrent uterine prolapse was seen. All women engage in sexual intercourse; in four women, six children have been delivered by caesarean section. One of these women, with an incontinent epispadias and sling plasty, developed a slight uterine prolapse during pregnancy. As urinary diversion, two have an ileocaecal pouch with continent umbilical stoma (three pregnancies) and one had a colon conduit (two pregnancies) which was recently integrated in a sigma–rectum pouch at her request for continence. Five women currently want to bear children.

All men, apart from one who had necrosis of the penis after primary bladder closure performed at an outside hospital, achieve erection. Of the 32 men with genital reconstruction, 11 have penile deviation, which is distressing in only two. Only two of the men are dissatisfied with the cosmetic result. In 28%, epididymitis occurred, necessitating orchiectomy (two) or vasectomy (three).

No patient with reconstruction of the external genitalia can ejaculate normally or has fathered children, whereas all five who did not undergo genital reconstruction had normal ejaculation and two have fathered a total of four children. Two of these five men underwent subsequent reconstruction, followed by urethral strictures and loss of ejaculation.

Discussion

Primary bladder closure up to 72 h after birth followed by bladder neck reconstruction (Young–Dees) at the age of $2^1/_2$ to 5 years is still the gold standard in the treatment of bladder exstrophy at most institutions.[18] Reimplantation of the ureters and additional pelvic osteotomy is often performed. The continence rate is up to 80% and, in well-selected patients, even higher.[6] However, multiple reoperations are often required to achieve continence.[19]

The term continence, as it concerns bladder closure, appears to be defined in different ways.[5,7,8] Jones et al.[7] define totally dry as continent day and night for more than 4 h wearing regular underclothes without need of incontinence pads. They achieved complete continence with the standard Young–Dees–Leadbetter bladder neck repair in 39%, with a modification in 64% of the patients. Jeffs reported, at the meeting of the American Academy of Pediatric Urology in 1992, that in their group of 5- to 10-year-old patients only 20% were completely dry.[20] Encouraged by the worldwide trend in the 1980s, the authors performed a Young–Dees procedure and Mainz pouch augmentation in nine patients, but the results were disappointing: five patients have needed conversion to a Mainz pouch I and only two patients with follow-up are continent day and night; however, the residual urine in one is about 40 ml.

One reason for failure of bladder closure and bladder neck reconstruction is that the creation of a functional sphincter mechanism is extremely difficult, in fact most impossible. To achieve continence, additional procedures beyond a Young–Dees–Leadbetter bladder neck reconstruction are often necessary and include intestinal bladder augmentation, pubovaginal sling, artificial urinary sphincter replacement and ureter reimplantation.[19]

A further reason for failure of bladder reconstruction is the detrusor muscle itself. Urodynamic studies of Hollowell et al.[21] demonstrated urine leakage due to involuntary detrusor contractions in ten of 18 patients with an unsatisfactory state of continence. In the continent group, five of seven patients could not void effectively and required CIC to empty the bladder completely. Only two of 25 patients investigated (8%) demonstrated normal bladder behaviour during filling and contractile voiding. The authors concluded that 'evolution to completely normal lower urinary tract function after bladder neck reconstruction is an unrealistic expectation for the majority of children with exstrophy and severe epispadias'.[21]

Nevertheless, the achievement of continence and preservation of the upper urinary tract must be the main goals. Mesrobian et al.[8] showed that hydronephrosis (25%) and reflux (43%) are common in patients with primary bladder closure, and thus could lead to deterioration of renal function.[8] The alternative to primary bladder closure is urinary diversion.

Ureterosigmoidostomy was the first form of continent urinary diversion.[22] After initial enthusiasm in the first half of the century, a high postoperative complication rate occurred and deterioration of the upper urinary tract became evident. Electrolyte imbalance, urinary tract infection, pyelonephritis, renal insufficiency and uraemia were not uncommon in the past.[8,23] An increasing number of colon tumours in ureterosigmoidostomy also reduced the frequency of this operation. Refinements of the operative techniques in ureterosigmoidostomy, antireflux ureteral implantation, improved antibiotics and also suture materials, make this standard surgical procedure a good alternative form of continent urinary diversion. A previously dilated upper urinary tract is a contraindication, as the authors have learned. Incontinence is mainly associated with late urinary diversion.[24,25] Upon entering school, 93% of the authors' children, with primary ureterosigmoidostomy performed before the age of 6, are completely continent.

The sigma rectum pouch (Mainz pouch II), a modification of ureterosigmoidostomy, offers some advantages. The fixation of the rectosigmoid junction at the promontory, as well as parallel ureteral implantations, guarantees a straight ureteral path and obviates kinking and subsequent obstruction. The antimesenteric opening of the bowel creates a low-pressure reservoir, precluding reflux and subsequent pyelonephritis.[11] This is the prerequisite for good continence and for avoidance of pyelonephritis or dilatation of the upper urinary tract. Two of the three reimplantations in our patients were necessitated by obstructive hyperplastic polyps. This high rate of ureter reimplantation (19%) conflicts with the rate of 7% in all 73 patients with Mainz pouch II, but the reason for this is not clear; however, no conversion to another type of urinary diversion was necessary in any patient.

For patients with complete incontinence, unsuccessful biofeedback training and medical treatment, as well as a low anal sphincter pressure, the authors recommend the Mainz pouch I. This continent urinary diversion is created as a low-pressure reservoir with a high capacity.[26] In four patients the previously constructed ileal or colon conduits were integrated into the reservoir to avoid metabolic disturbance on removing too much bowel.

Intermediary forms of urinary diversion, especially the colon conduit, should be used in individuals with a dilated urinary upper tract and the risk of renal insufficiency. It provides the advantage of a low pressure system, leading to stabilization or recovery of renal function.[12]

Patients with bladder exstrophy have a risk of secondary malignancies.[8] Most reports in the literature concern ureterosigmoidostomy; however, it should be remembered that it is the oldest type of urinary diversion and many patients have a long-term follow-up. The risk of colon carcinoma after ureterosigmoidostomy has been calculated as about 5%;[27,28] this is about 150–500 times higher than that of the normal population but does not evaluate the operative technique nor the geographically racially correlated incidence of colon carcinoma.[27–29] Thus screening is mandatory: colonoscopy must be performed 5 years after ureterosigmoidostomy and repeated annually. After a mean follow-up of 18.8 years in the 32 reported patients with ureterosigmoidostomy, not one neoplasm has occurred. However, all patients with bowel segments used for urinary tract reconstruction are at risk of secondary malignancies.[30] If malignancy is detected at an early stage by biopsy, conversion from a continent rectal reservoir to a Mainz pouch I with continent umbilical stoma is the authors' method of choice.

The cosmetic results after approximation of the clitoris and mons pubis as well as reconstruction of the labia minora are good. However, after vaginoplasty, uterine prolapse may occur.[2,13] There are only a few reports in the literature regarding the treatment of uterine prolapse in patients with bladder exstrophy.[3,31–33] In 1956, Overstreet and Hinman[33] used two lateral fascial strips attached to the anterior surface of the uterine cornu; additionally, the anterior cervical wall was fixed to the anterior abdominal wall. Woodhouse used a Gore-tex® (polytetrafluoroethylene) sling, sutured to the promontory after mobilization of the rectum and wrapped around the uterus at the level of the cervix.[3] Dewhurst et al.[31] used an Ivalon sponge hysterosacropexy in two patients. In women with suspicion of prolapse or after prolapse, the authors carry out antefixation of the uterus, which permits individual adaptation to different anatomical situations caused by the varying distance between the pubic bones. Additional fixation of the uterus to the ligament between the pubic bones results in enlargement of the vagina.[34]

Fertility in females is normal. In a recently published series of four pregnancies after orthotopic continent urinary diversion (Indiana pouch) with perineal stoma, all four women developed uterine prolapse and urinary tract infections, two developed hydronephrosis and two had difficulty with CIC.[35] In contrast, two of the reported patients with ileocaecal pouch and continent umbilical stoma suffered no complications.

Reconstruction of the external genitalia and urethra of male patients is technically more complex and associated with a higher rate of complications. The cosmetic results are good: even if the penis still deviates — an unsatisfactory result for the surgeon — the patient may be thoroughly satisfied with the function. The most serious late complication, however, is iatrogenic infertility.[36] In patients with urinary diversion, construction of an infrapubic opening to a small reservoir above the verumontanum at the penile base offers the advantage of being able to aspirate sperm easily. None of the authors' patients treated in this way had subsequent epididymitis.

Conclusions

Body image and freedom of lifestyle are improved by eliminating an external collection device. These two points become very important in adolescent patients in particular. Currently, the main indication for urinary conversion is the wish of the patient for continence. However, every new intervention is accompanied by high risk of complications and failures. The risk and the realistic advantages must be explained to the patient. The conversion operation should be performed at a specialized centre by a surgeon who is familiar with the various types of urinary diversion.

Patients with continent forms of urinary diversion are continent day and night, in general. This is the standard that reconstructive surgery of primary bladder closure must attain; however, in view of the results of urodynamic studies, this seems to be a rather vain hope in patients with primary bladder closure.[21]

Reconstruction of the external and internal genitalia in women creates good cosmetic results; however, the risk of uterine prolapse should always be kept in mind. Fertility is not problematic, even in women with urinary diversions. However, the risk of infertility after genital reconstruction in male patients is extremely high.

References

1. Lancaster P A L. Epidemiology of bladder exstrophy and epispadias: a communication from the international clearinghouse for birth defects monitoring systems. Teratology 1987; 36: 221–227
2. Burbige K A, Hensle T W, Chambers W J et al. Pregnancy and sexual function in women with bladder exstrophy. Urology 1986; 28: 12–14
3. Woodhouse C R J. Exstrophy and epispadias. In: Woodhouse C R J (ed) Long-term paediatric urology, 1st ed. Oxford: Blackwell Scientific Publications, 1991: 127–150
4. Ansell J S. Surgical treatment of exstrophy in bladder with emphasis on neonatal primary closure. J Urol 1979; 121: 650–653
5. Gearhart J P, Jeffs R D. Exstrophy of the bladder, epispadias and other bladder anomalies. In: Walsh P C, Retik A B, Stamey T A, Vaughan E D (eds) Campbell's Urology, 6th ed. New York: Saunders, 1992: 1772–1821
6. Husman D A, McLorie G A, Churchill B M. Closure of the exstrophic bladder. J Urol 1989; 142: 522–524
7. Jones J A, Mitchell M E, Rink R C. Improved results using a modification of the Young–Dees–Leadbetter bladder neck repair. Br J Urol 1993; 71: 555–561
8. Mesrobian H-G J, Kelalis P P, Kramer S A. Long-term follow-up of 103 patients with bladder exstrophy. J Urol 1988; 139: 719–722
9. Stöckle M, Becht E, Voges G et al. Ureterosigmoidostomy: an outdated approach to bladder exstrophy? J Urol 1990; 143: 770–775
10. Zabbo A, Kay R. Ureterosigmoidostomy and bladder exstrophy: a long term follow-up. J Urol 1986; 136: 396–398
11. Fisch M, Wammack R, Müller S C, Hohenfellner R. Mainz Pouch II (Sigma rectum pouch). J Urol 1993; 149: 258–264
12. Richie J P, Skinner D G. Urinary diversion: the physiological rationale for colonic conduits. Br J Urol 1975; 47: 269–275
13. Krisiloff M, Puchner P J, Tretter W et al. Pregnancy in women with bladder exstrophy. J Urol 1978; 119: 478–479
14. Blakeley C R, Mills W G. The obstetric and gynaecological complications of bladder exstrophy and epispadias. Br J Obstet Gynaecol 1981; 88: 167–173
15. Lepor H, Sharpio E, Jeffs R D. Urethral reconstruction in boys with classical bladder exstrophy. J Urol 1984; 131: 512–515
16. Mellin Y, Lottmann H, Cendron J. Genito-sexual outcome of patients treated for bladder exstrophy. Proc Eur Soc Ped Urol 1992 (abstr 123)
17. Käser O, Iklé F A. Abdominale Operationen bei Lageveränderungen des Genitales. In: Käser O, Iklé F A (eds) Operationen in der Gynäkologie. Stuttgart: Thieme, 1982: 1–10

18. Gearhart J P. Editorial comments. J Urol 1990; 143: 774

19. Connor J P, Hensle T W, Lattimer J K, Burbige K A. Long-term follow-up of 207 patients with bladder exstrophy: an evolution in treatment. J Urol 1989; 142: 793–796

20. Jeffs R D. Discussion at the AAP 1992, San Francisco. J Urol 1993; 150: 634

21. Hollowell J G, Hill P D, Duffy P G, Ransley P G. Evaluation and treatment of incontinence after bladder neck reconstruction in exstrophy and epispadias. Br J Urol 1993; 71: 743–749

22. Simon J. Ectopia vesica (absence of the anterior walls of the bladder and pubic abdominal parieties) operation for directing the orifices of the ureters into the rectum: temporary success; subsequent death; autopsy. Lancet 1852; 2: 736

23. Bennett A H. Exstrophy of bladder treated by ureterosigmoidostomies: long-term evaluation. Urology 1973; 2: 165–168

24. Silverman S H, Woodhouse C R J, Strachan J R et al. Long-term management of patients who have had urinary diversion into colon. Br J Urol 1986; 58: 634–639

25. Macfarlane M T, Lattimer J K, Hensle T W. The unheralded hazard of ureterosigmoidostomy. Pediatrics 1976; 64: 668–671

26. Thüroff J W, Alken P, Riedmiller H et al. 100 cases of Mainz Pouch: continuing experience and evolution. J Urol 1988; 140: 283–288

27. Pierce E H Jr, Zickermann P, Leadbetter G W Jr. Ureterosigmoidostomy and carcinoma of the colon. Trans Am Assoc Genito-Urin Surg 1978; 70: 92–94

28. Sooriyaarachchi G S, Johnson R O, Carbone P P. Neoplasm of the large bowel following ureterosigmoidostomy. Arch Surg 1977; 112: 1174–1179

29. Spence H M, Hoffmann W W, Fosmire G P. Tumors of the colon as a late complication of ureterosigmoidostomy for exstrophy of the bladder. Br J Urol 1979; 51: 446–470

30. Kälble T, Schreiber W, Berger M R et al. Karzinomrisiko in verschiedenen Formen der Harnableitung unter Verwendung von Darm. Aktuel Urol 1993; 24: 1–7

31. Dewhurst J, Toplis P J, Shepherd J H. Ivalon sponge hysterosacropexy for genital prolapse in patients with bladder exstrophy. Br J Obstet Gynaecol 1980; 87: 67–69

32. Mariona F G, Evans T N. Pregnancy following repair of anal and vaginal atresia and bladder exstrophy. Obstet Gynecol 1982; 59: 653–654

33. Overstreet E W, Hinman F Jr. Some gynaecologic aspects of bladder exstrophy. West J Surg Obstet Gynecol 1956; 64: 131–137

34. Stein R, Fisch M, Schumacher S et al. Operative Korrektur des äußeren und inneren weiblichen Genitale bei Blasenekstrophie. Aktuel Urol Op Tech 1994; 25: I–XI

35. Kennedy W A, Hensle T W, Reiley E A et al. Pregnancy after orthotopic continent urinary diversion. Surg Gynecol Obstet 1993; 177: 405–409

36. Stein R, Stöckle M, Fisch M et al. The fate of the adult exstrophy patient. J Urol 1994; 152: 1413–1416

Continent gastric urinary reservoirs in paediatric patients

15

J. R. Woodard   R. Gosalbez
T. S. Parrott   L. M. Pérez
B. H. Broecker   C. A. Massad

Introduction

The use of various intestinal segments in the reconstruction of the lower urinary tract began in 1851 when Simon performed bilateral ureteroproctostomies in a 13-year-old boy born with bladder exstrophy.[1] Each segment of bowel has advantages and disadvantages and none is clearly superior. Metabolic disturbances, mucus production, altered nutrition and developmental growth, reservoir perforation, and carcinogenesis have been well documented with the use of jejunum, ileum, and right and left colon.[2] Although Sinaiko first used a gastric segment for the construction of a urinary conduit in 1956, it was not until recently that the gastric segment became popular, mainly through the reports of Leong and Mitchell.[2–6] Although much has been written by these authors concerning gastric neobladders and gastrocystoplasties, few objective data have been presented concerning continent gastric reservoirs. This chapter reports the authors' experience with 22 patients over the last 3 years who underwent construction of continent gastric reservoirs.

Patients and methods

Between January 1991 and February 1994, a total of 22 patients (eight male and 14 female) underwent some form of continent gastric urinary diversion at the authors' institutions. Patient ages ranged from 4 to 25 (mean 11) years. The indication for operation in all patients was urinary incontinence refractory to more conservative forms of management. Table 15.1 lists the congenital disorders that caused the incontinence. All patients with bladder exstrophy had undergone bladder closure and those with classic bladder exstrophy at least one type of bladder neck

Diagnosis	No. of patients
Meningomyelocoele	4
Exstrophy–epispadias complex	7*
Cloacal exstrophy	7†
Cloacal malformation	2
Rhabdomyosarcoma of prostate	1
Neurofibromatosis	1

*One patient had spinal dysraphism and a sacrococcygeal teratoma at birth.
†Three patients had meningomyelocoeles, one had sacral agenesis and one occult spinal dysraphism.

Table 15.1. Indications for urinary diversion

reconstruction. One patient had a solitary kidney and five patients had one kidney with differential function of less than 30% of total renal function. One of these latter patients underwent simultaneous nephroureterectomy. Two other patients had suffered acute renal failure in the past (one requiring temporary dialysis), with normalization of serum creatinine by the time of gastric reservoir reconstruction.

The gastric reservoir was the first form of urinary diversion for 11 patients; it was a secondary form of diversion of the other 11 who previously had intestinal urinary conduits (four ileal and two sigmoid colon), enterocystoplasties (one sigmoid and one right colon), vesicostomy (two), and bilateral cutaneous ureterostomies (one).

In five patients the reservoir was made entirely of stomach (group I), while in ten others a gastrocystoplasty was performed with surgical closure of the bladder neck (group II). Two of the group II patients had gastric augmentation of already existing colonic cystoplasties (one sigmoid and one ileocaecal). In seven additional patients a composite gastrointestinal continent reservoir was created using the detubularized existing bowel conduits in six (four ileal and two sigmoid) and a fresh segment of ileum in one other patient (group III).

A wedge of the gastric greater curvature based on either the right (20) or left (two) gastroepiploic artery pedicle was isolated, as previously described by Mitchell and associates using the gastrointestinal anastomosis (GIA) stapler (90 mm).[2] A total of 26 ureters in 16 patients were reimplanted in an antireflux fashion (11 ureters into the bladder, nine into the gastric reservoir, and six ureters through three intussuscepted ileal nipples). In one patient with an ileocaecal augmentation cystoplasty performed at an outside institution, an intussuscepted ileocaecal valve was used as the antireflux mechanism. While four patients underwent transureteroureterostomy (TUU) at the time of gastric reservoir reconstruction, one patient had had a previous TUU. Another patient with a pelvic kidney underwent a pyeloureterostomy.

The Mitrofanoff principle was the continence mechanism in all patients. The appendix was used in eight patients, ureter in six, a gastric augment and single pedicle (GASP) tube in four,[7] tapered ileum in three, and tapered sigmoid in one patient. The catheterizable stoma was created at the umbilicus in nine patients, in the lower abdominal quadrant in ten (right in seven, left in three), and in the pubic region in three patients using ureter on an isolated vascular pedicle.

Results

With a follow-up of 6–38 (mean 24) months no deaths have occurred. Postoperative complications have occurred in 15 of the authors' 22 patients and are listed in Table 15.2. An early complication occurred in the first patient, who suffered a left subphrenic abcess requiring surgical intervention following unsuccessful percutaneous drainage. No patient in this series has suffered from the haematuria and dysuria syndrome.[8] One patient receiving postoperative total parenteral alimentation developed

Complications	No. of patients*		
	Group I (n = 5)	Group II (n = 10)	Group III (n = 7)
Hypochloraemic hypokalaemic metabolic alkalosis	1	3[†]	1
Peristomal abcess	–	1	–
Reservoir–cutaneous fistula	–	2	–
Bowel obstruction, enterocutaneous fistula, incontinent ileal Mitrofanoff	1	–	–
Left subphrenic abcess, ureterogastric anastomotic stricture	1	–	–
Recurrent UTI	1	–	1
Pyelonephritis	–	–	2
Angulated gastric Mitrofanoff	–	–	1
Fungal sepsis	–	–	1

*Group I, complete gastric reservoir; group II, gastrocystoplasty, closed bladder neck; group III, composite reservoir
[†]One patient required two hospitalizations.

Table 15.2. Postoperative complications

fungal sepis (*Candida albicans*). Another patient required open exploration 3 days after reservoir activation, because of inability to catheterize a GASP tube Mitrofanoff: an open procedure was required, owing to an acute angulation that was easily corrected with lysis of adhesions, without having to take down the stoma itself.

Continence

Of the 22 patients, 21 were completely continent at early and last follow-up on a self-catheterization programme of every 3–4 h. In one patient, a 6-year-old girl with cloacal exstrophy, there was an incompetent tapered ileal Mitrofanoff mechanism of the gastric reservoir. Her course was complicated by bowel obstruction requiring exploration 5 weeks postoperatively, before activation of her reservoir. This in turn was complicated by enterocutaneous fistulas requiring total perenteral nutrition. She underwent surgical revision 1 year later, when her only remaining enterocutaneous fistula was closed, the ileal Mitrofanoff reservoir was removed and a hemi-Koch augmentation of the gastric reservoir (noted intraoperatively to be of small capacity) was undertaken. She is now continent with a stapled intussuscepted ileal nipple as her continence mechanism.

Video-urodynamics

All ten patients undergoing gastrocystoplasty underwent preoperative video-urodynamic studies. So far 14 patients (three in group I, six in group II, and five in group III) have undergone video-urodynamics from 3 to 14 (mean 7) months postoperatively. The mean bladder capacity was 315 ml for group I, 340 ml for group II, and 360 ml for group III patients. Three of the 14 patients (two in group II and one in group III) had suboptimal compliance (10, 20 and 22 ml/cmH$_2$O). Bolus contractions (instability) with a pressure above 15 cmH$_2$O (range 28–48 cmH$_2$O) were present in five of the 14 patients. All leak-point pressures have been above 60 cmH$_2$O, with most above 100 cmH$_2$O. No significant reflux was detected postoperatively in any patient.

Renal function and metabolic disturbances

Renal function, as measured by serum creatinine, nuclear medicine renography and intravenous urography, improved or remained stable in all patients. Only one patient had deterioration of the upper tracts secondary to a partial ureterogastric anastomotic stricture, which developed 12 months postoperatively and required surgical revision.

Five patients of the 22 patients (23%) have required a total of six hospitalizations (each from 2 to 8 days) for hypochloraemic hypokalaemic metabolic alkalosis. All responded quickly to hydration with intravenous normal saline, catheter drainage and intravenous H_2 blockers. One patient, previously reported,[9] required arginine hydrochloride therapy for severe metabolic alkalosis following a bout of gastroenteritis 4 months postoperatively. Serum gastrin levels were elevated in three of the 22 patients (137, 145 and 168 pg/ml, normal 0–125); two of these three patients had bouts of hypochloraemic alkalosis. Although all patients are placed on H_2 blocker therapy for the first few weeks postoperatively, five of the 22 patients continue on such therapy at last follow-up.

Infections

Two patients (both with composite gastrointestinal reservoirs) have suffered pyelonephritis requiring short hospitalizations without recurrences. Two other patients have had occasional but recurrent urinary tract infections, with each episode responsive to oral antibiotics. (One with a total gastric reservoir and the other with a composite reservoir.) One patient with a ureteral Mitrofanoff developed a peristomal infection 16 months postoperatively and was successfully treated with catheter drainage and intravenous antibiotics for 3 days. The same patient experienced spontaneous urinary drainage from her old suprapubic tube site 36 months postoperatively which healed with 3 weeks of catheter drainage and antibiotics.

Discussion

In 1956, Edwin Sinaiko of Chicago was perhaps the first to use a wedge of stomach in order to construct a gastric conduit.[3] The stoma of the first gastric conduit was managed with a permanent catheter placed in the pouch. Sinaiko learned from this first case and subsequently improved his technique when he created the second gastric conduit in 1958.[10] He isolated a portion of the gastric fundus along the greater curvature, its vasculature based on the right gastroepiploic artery. The stoma was placed within the existing paramedian incision at the level of the umbilicus. In 1978, Leong of Hong Kong reported the successful creation of a gastric conduit in 21 patients.[5] Following a significant experience with gastric neobladders and gastrocystoplasties, rather than using a wedge (as Sinaiko had done), Leong used the whole gastric pyloric antrum based on the left gastroepiploic artery, and brought it through an opening in the transverse mesocolon, with the stoma placed in the right iliac fossa. In 1977, Rudick and associates of New York developed a continent urinary reservoir using stomach in dogs.[11] They constructed a pouch using a large wedge of gastric fundus and created a continent stoma by using a modification of the Janeway–Depage tubovalvular gastrostomy. Although the initial capacity of the reservoir was approximately 200 ml, by 2 weeks postoperatively the pouch retained over 1 litre remaining completely continent for 6 months. More recently, Mitchell and associates have popularized the use of a gastric wedge in the reconstruction of the urinary tract and have constructed at least three completely continent reservoirs.[6,8] Others have used composite urinary reservoirs in which a segment of stomach and either colon or ileum are joined for a more voluminous and compliant reservoir.[12,13]

The authors have previously reported their experience with the use of the stomach in urinary reconstruction.[7,9,14] Clearly, their early experience, as well as that of others, suggests that the use of stomach has advantages for patients with renal insufficiency or short bowel conditions. It also has the advantage of decreased mucus production compared with ileum or large bowel, a fact that is particularly attractive for reconstructions in children who self-catheterize with smaller catheters. Moreover, the stomach allows for easy submucosal tunnelling for antireflux ureteral reimplantation, the Mitrofanoff technique and the recently reported GASP tube catheterizable stoma.[7] However, the use of a gastric segment in the urinary tract is not free from problems: these include the dysuria–haematuria syndrome and hypochloraemic hypokalaemic metabolic alkalosis requiring long-term therapy with H_2 blockers, and are unpredictable as to when and in whom they may occur. None of the authors' patients with continent gastric reservoirs have suffered from dysuria–haematuria syndrome, which the authors have clearly seen in those patients with gastrocystoplasties who catheterize through the urethra. On the other hand, it appears that a larger proportion of patients (23% in the authors' series) with a continent gastric reservoir suffer from metabolic alkalosis. This latter disturbance, in most cases, is easily treated with intravenous normal saline hydration, catheter drainage and H_2 blockers.[9]

The continence achieved by the Mitrofanoff procedure in the gastric reservoir has been extremely satisfying. Video-urodynamic studies conducted at an early stage of follow-up have revealed a reasonably capacious and compliant reservoir in most cases. Although all reservoirs were found to have a high leak-point pressure (most being more than 100 cmH_2O), no deterioration of upper tracts has been documented. This fact stresses the requirement for all ureters to have an adequate antireflux mechanism as well as the need for close radiological follow-up. Cystometry at an early stage has suggested that totally gastric reservoirs have the lowest capacity. It will be important to determine whether such is the case on longer follow-up studies.

Although one of the advantages of the use of the stomach is its alleged lower incidence of bacteriuria and urinary tract infections, it is not totally free from these problems, as two of the authors' patients required hospitalization for pyelonephritis and two others have recurrent urinary tract infections (one occurring in a totally gastric reservoir, the other three occurring in composite gastrointestinal reservoirs).

In conclusion, although it is not without complications, the continent gastric reservoir in its various configurations is an important addition to the armamentarium of the reconstructive urologist, for properly selected patients.

References

1. Simon J. Extropia vesicae (absence of the anterior walls of the bladder and pubic abdominal parieties): operation for directing the orifices of the ureters into the rectum: temporary success; subsequent death; autopsy. Lancet 1852; 2: 568–569
2. Nguyen D H, Mitchell M E. Gastric bladder reconstruction. Urol Clin North Am 1991; 18: 649–657
3. Sinaiko E S. Artificial bladder in man from segment of stomach. Surg Forum 1957; 8: 635
4. Leong C H, Ong G B. Gastrocystoplasty in dogs. Aust NZ J Surg 1972; 41: 272–279
5. Leong C H. Use of the stomach for bladder replacement and urinary diversion. Ann R Coll Surg Engl 1978; 60: 283–289
6. Nguyen D H, Ganesan G S, Mitchell M E. Lower urinary tract reconstruction using stomach tissue in children and young adults. World J Urol 1992; 10: 76
7. Gosalbez R, Padron O F, Singla A K et al. The gastric augment single pedicle tube catheterizable stoma: a useful adjunct to reconstruction of the urinary tract. J Urol 152 (October 1994-in press).
8. Nguyen D H, Bain M A, Salmonson K L et al. The syndrome of dysuria and hematuria in pediatric urinary reconstruction with stomach. J Urol 1993; 150: 707–709
9. Gosalbez R, Woodard J R, Broecker B H, Warshaw B. Metabolic complications of the use of the use of stomach for urinary reconstruction. J Urol 1993; 150: 710–712
10. Sinaiko E S. Artificial bladder from a gastric pouch. Surg Gynecol Obstet 1960; 111: 155
11. Rudick J, Schonholz S, Weber H B. The gastric bladder: a continent reservoir for urinary diversion. Surgery 1977; 82: 1
12. Bihrle R, Foster R S, Steidle C P et al. Creation of a transverse colon–gastric composite reservoir: a new technique. J Urol 1989; 141: 1217
13. Lockhart J L, Davies R, Cox C et al. The gastroileoileal pouch: an alternative continent urinary reservoir for patients with short bowel acidosis and/or extensive pelvic radiation. J Urol 1993; 150: 46–50
14. Gosalbez R, Woodard J R, Broecker B H et al. The use of stomach in pediatric urinary reconstruction. J Urol 1993; 150: 438–440

16

Ileocaecal valve reconstruction during continent urinary diversion

M. Fisch   F. Spies   R. Wammack
R. Bürger   R. Hohenfellner

Introduction

In the course of several procedures that are currently favoured for continent urinary diversion (Mainz pouch;[1] Indiana Pouch[2]), the ileocaecal valve is destroyed. Bearing in mind the two main functions of the ileocaecal valve (prolongation of intestinal transit time and prevention of colo–ileal reflux),[3,4] it seems plausible that resection of the valve in certain patients may aggravate or induce diarrhoea or symptoms similar to the short bowel syndrome. Patients who previously have undergone extensive bowel resection or irradiation seem to be particularly at risk. Children with anal atresia in association with urogenital malformations or myelomeningocoele, and who have already experienced diarrhoea preoperatively, may suffer from severe diarrhoea and frequency of stools after urinary diversion and subsequent loss of the ileocaecal valve.[5] Whether this is attributable solely to the lack of transit time prolongation, or absorption anomalies secondary to bacterial colonization of the ileum are responsible, is a matter of debate.[4]

In view of their experience with the submucosally embedded appendix as a continence mechanism in continent urinary diversion,[6] the authors have attempted to apply this technique to the reconstruction of the ileocaecal valve.

Surgical technique

After the ileocaecal segment has been isolated the ascending colon is closed by single-stitch seromuscular polyglyconate 4/0 sutures. Subsequently, the taenia libera of the ascending colon is incised longitudinally over a length of 6–7 cm, starting 1 cm above the closed end. By dissecting the muscular layer from the mucosa, as for submucosal embedding of the appendix during continent urinary diversion,[6] a broad trough is created for the ileum. This dissection of the seromuscular layer from the mucosa can easily be accomplished by blunt dissection using a 'peanut'.

At the cranial end, a 2 cm incision is made in the mucosa for the anastomosis of the ileal loop. The ileum is incised antimesenterically to obtain a large entrance without obstruction. The preparation of the ileal mesentery is of the utmost importance in order that the blood supply of the embedded segment is not compromised. The mesentery is defatted and the serosa removed, as for preparation of the mesentery in order to create an invaginated ileal nipple during the Mainz pouch I continent urinary diversion.[1] An ileocaecal anastomosis, grasping all layers of the ileum and the mucosa of the colon (Fig. 16.1) is then created, using single-stitch polyglyconate 5/0 sutures. Subsequently, the seromuscular layer is closed over the anastomosed ileal segment, thus creating a submucosal tunnel 4 cm in length. Lateral adaptation stitches allow the ileum to dive smoothly into the caecum and avoid mucosal diverticula or kinking and obstruction (Fig. 16.2).

Clinical results

At the time of writing, the authors have conducted this operation in 30 patients. Indications for reconstruction of the ileocaecal valve were previous irradiation, extensive bowel resection, an incompetent anal

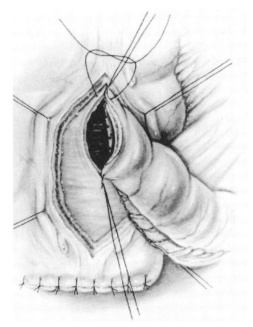

Figure 16.1. Ascending colon closed terminally, taenia libera incised and seromuscular layer dissected bluntly from mucosa. Colonic mucosa is incised for ileocaecal anastomosis.

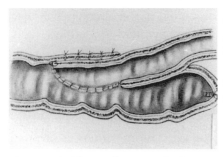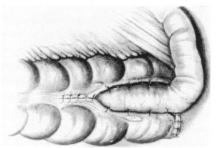

Figure 16.2. Closure of seromuscular layer to create a submucosal tunnel 4 cm in length (left). The lateral view (right) shows the ileum diving smoothly into the caecum, avoiding mucosal diverticula or kinking and obstruction.

sphincter or diarrhoea (Table 16.1). The underlying aetiology was myelomeningocoele or neurogenic bladder disturbances in 16 patients, malignancy in seven, congenital anomalies in six patients and trauma in one patient.

No intraoperative complications were encountered. In one patient (3.3%) a relaparotomy had to be performed, owing to bowel obstruction, and the reconstructed ileocaecal valve was resected. In the remaining 29 cases the postoperative course was uneventful. Of the 30 patients, 26 were followed (mean follow-up 15.2 months, range 2–29 months). Three patients left the country and were thus lost to follow-up and one is still in the immediate postoperative period. One patient died of malignancy (gynaecological cancer) 15 months after surgery.

The preoperatively existing stool frequency was maintained or even reduced postoperatively in the majority of patients (81%), even though a considerable amount of bowel was removed during the urinary diversion procedure (Table 16.2).

Indication	No. of patients
Extensive bowel resection	9
Incompetent anal sphincter	12
Irradiation	4
Diarrhoea	8
Total	33*

*In four patients there was more than one indication.

Table 16.1. Indications for reconstruction of the ileocaecal valve in 29 patients

Period	Stool frequency/type	No. of patients
Preoperative	1–2 /day	12
	>2/day	6
	Constipation	5
	Constipation and diarrhoea	3
Postoperative	Frequency reduced	7
	Frequency maintained	14
	Frequency increased	5

Table 16.2. Preoperative stool type and frequency and postoperative change in frequency, after reconstruction of the ileocaecal valve during continent urinary diversion

Discussion

Whereas the metabolic consequences of bowel resection and of the use of intestine for urinary diversion have been the subject of numerous studies, little attention has been paid to the effects of bowel resection on lower gastrointestinal symptoms. Severe diarrhoea is an unusual consequence of urinary diversion in patients without a history of bowel resection or irradiation, but mild changes in bowel function seem to be more common than expected. Mark and coworkers[7] reviewed 253 patients who had previously undergone augmentation, substitution or replacement cystoplasty in order to determine postoperative bowel dysfunction. They found alterations in bowel function in 29% of patients, 69 of whom described long-term symptoms (mild in 37, moderate in 25 and severe in seven). Risk factors were patients with neurological illness and those with interstitial cystitis, resection of the ileocaecal valve, previous bowel symptoms, and removal of more than 40 cm of small intestine in patients with neurogenic bladder.

From a metabolic point of view, resection of the proximal small bowel is tolerated better than resection of the distal small bowel.[8] Moreover, when removal of the ileocaecal valve and right colectomy are associated with extensive bowel resection, water and electrolyte diarrhoea are significantly greater and steatorrhoea is more severe and prolonged.[8] In a group of 25 patients after bowel resection, Mitchell et al.[9] demonstrated that diarrhoea was worse in patients who had lost the ileocaecal valve and part of the right colon than in patients after resection of a comparable ileal segment. Reconstruction of the ileocaecal valve can obviate diarrhoea or a further increase in frequency of stools in selected patients.

Various surgical techniques have been employed in an attempt to prolong gastrointestinal transit time: these include incorporation of reverse segments,[10-13] bowel intussusception,[14] myectomy[15,16] and, ultimately, reconstruction of the ileocaecal valve.[17-21] Most of these procedures have been carried out on an experimental basis in dogs[14,22] or rats;[23] only very occasionally has such a procedure been performed in humans.[10-14]

The use of an isoperistaltic segment was common practice in the 1950s and 1960s. Although increasing transit time, however, the reversed segments did not improve absorptive deficiencies, yet produced a significant complication rate (obstruction and anastomotic disruption).[4,14,16,22] In addition, they exacerbated bacteriological contamination of the remaining small bowel.[15] Equally, ileo–ileal intussusception frequently resulted in obstruction.[14]

Myectomies of the small intestinal wall have been classified as partial and total.[15] In the former, the circular muscular layer is removed; in the latter, both the circular and the longitudinal layers are resected, keeping the mucosal wall intact. Total myectomies, keeping the free borders of the incision apart, lead to formation of mucosal diverticula. If the borders are sutured, a mucosal valve is created. The reduction of transit time was probably achieved by a reduction of the lumen by the infolding of the mucosa.[17-20] Other techniques, such as invagination of the small bowel into the large bowel or vice versa, have been reported; however, they have had only modest success.[14] None of the procedures described has been widely accepted, because of the high rate of complications and doubtful clinical benefit.

In 1984, Vinograd and coworkers[21] tried to apply the concept of the submucosal tunnel, for ureteral neoimplantation into the bladder, to the gastrointestinal tract in order to create an artificial valve. After bowel resection he incised the serosa and muscularis mucosa circumferentially at two points, leaving only the colonic mucosa intact. A plane over the colonic mucosa and under the muscularis mucosae was formed by blunt dissection, thus creating a submucosal tunnel. The colonic mucosa was opened at the end of the tunnel and a two-layer anastomosis created. Tunnel lengths of 2, 4 and 6 cm were used. None of the 25 dogs with reconstructed ileocaecal valves showed obstruction. Vinograd found a fourfold delay in transit time in these dogs, compared with controls with a simple end-to-end anastomosis. A tunnel length of 4 cm was sufficient to prevent caeco–ileal reflux.

The results of extensive experiments in dogs, and the success of this operation in an animal model as well as in an initial group of patients, indicate that ileocaecal valve reconstruction can be accomplished by a simple and less complication-prone technique than previously practised. The operative technique is easily reproducible and has a short learning curve, as it is analogous to the Lich–Gregoir technique[24,25] for ureteral neoimplantation and to the Mainz pouch technique for submucosal embedding of the appendix during continent diversion.[6]

Simplicity, reproducibility and standardization, together with precise selection of patients liable to profit from this operation, will make ileocaecal valve reconstruction a most beneficial supplement to continent urinary diversion.

References

1. Thüroff J W, Alken P, Riedmiller H et al. 100 cases of Mainz Pouch: Continuing experience and evaluation. J Urol 1988; 140: 283–288
2. Rowland R G, Mitchell M E, Bihrle R et al. Indiana continent urinary reservoir. J Urol 1987; 137: 1136–1139
3. Singleton A O Jr, Redmond C II, McMurray E. Ileocecal resection and small bowel transit and absorption. Ann Surg 1964; 159: 690–693
4. Richardson J D, Griffen W O Jr. Ileocecal valve substitutes as bacteriologic barriers. Am J Surg 1972; 123: 149–153
5. Lie H R, Lagergren J, Rasmussen F et al. Bowel and bladder control of children with myelomeningocele: a Nordic study. Dev Med Child Neurol 1991; 33: 1053–1061
6. Riedmiller H, Bürger R, Müller S C et al. Continent appendix stoma: a modification of the Mainz pouch technique. J Urol 1990; 143: 1115–1117
7. Mark S D, MacDiarmid S A, Webster G D. Factors associated with bowel dysfunction following cystoplasty: analysis of 253 patients. J Urol 1993; 149: 370A
8. Cosnes J, Gendre J P, LeQuintrec Y. Role of the ileocecal valve and site of intestinal resection in malabsorption after extensive small bowel resection. Digestion 1978; 18: 329–335
9. Mitchell J E, Breuer R I, Zuckermann L et al. The colon influences ileal resection diarrhoea. Dig Dis Sci 1980; 25: 33–41
10. Gibson L D, Carter R, Hinshaw D B. Segmental reversal of small intestine after massive bowel resection. JAMA 1962; 182: 952–954
11. Madding G F, Kennedy P A, McLaughlin R T. Clinical use of antiperistaltic bowel segments. Ann Surg 1965; 161: 601–604
12. Shepard D. Antiperistaltic bowel segment in the treatment of short bowel syndrome. Ann Surg 1966; 163: 850–855
13. Venables C W, Ellis H, Smith A D M. Antiperistaltic segments after massive intestinal resection. Lancet 1966; 2: 1390–1394
14. Waddell W R, Kern F Jr, Halgrimson C G, Woodburgy J J. A simple jejunocolic 'valve'. Arch Surg 1970; 100: 438–444
15. Stacchini A, DiDio L J A, Primo L S et al. Artificial sphincters as surgical treatment for experimental massive resection of small intestine. Am J Surg 1982; 143: 721–726
16. Schiller W R, DiDio L J A, Anderson M C. Production of artificial sphincters. Ablation of the longitudinal layer of the intestine. Arch Surg 1967; 95: 436–442
17. Glassman J A. An artificial ileocecal valve. Surg Gynecol Obstet 1942; 74: 92–98
18. Ackroyd F W, Giles G, McDermott W V Jr. Ileal mucosal valve to prevent reflux at

the ileorectal anastomosis in the colon exclusion operation for hepatic encephalopathy. Surg Forum 1969; 20: 356–357

19. Blömer A, Dux A, Stobbe A et al. Operative Eingriffe zur Verlangsamung der Dünndarmpassage. Tierexperimentelle Untersuchungen. Langenbecks Arch Chir 1972; 330: 285–306

20. Hidalgo F, Lopez-Cortes M, Salas S J, Zavala J. Intestinal muscular layer ablation in short-bowel syndrome. Arch Surg 1973; 106: 188–190

21. Vinograd I, Merguerian P, Udassin R et al. An experimental model of a submucosally tunneled valve for the replacement of the ileocecal valve. J Pediatr Surg 1984; 19: 726–729

22. Ehtuish E F. The reverse of intestinal segments for the treatment of ileostomy diarrhoea. Acta Chir Iugosl 1989; 36: 239–249

23. Kinzel P, Wohlgemuth B, Schwokowski C F. Morphologische Veränderungen am Dünndarm nach experimenteller Resektion von 75% mittleren Dünndarms und passageverlangsamenden Operationsverfahren. Dtsch Z Verdau Stoffwechselkr 1988; 48: 94–103

24. Lich R, Howerton L, Davis L. Recurrent urosepsis in children. J Urol 1961; 86: 554–558

25. Gregoir W, Van Regenmorter G. Le reflux vésico-urétéral congénital. Urol Int 1964; 18: 122-136

Sigma–rectum pouch: a modification of ureterosigmoidostomy

17

M. Fisch   R. Wammack
R. Hohenfellner

Introduction

Ureterosigmoidostomy was the first form of continent urinary diversion.[1] During the first half of the 20th century the attendant high postoperative mortality and complication rate led to numerous modifications of the ureteral implantation technique.[2] By combination of a direct anastomosis of the ureter to the sigmoid colon with an antirefluxic submucosal tunnel, the rate of postoperative obstruction at the implantation site, as well as the rate of ascending infection, was significantly reduced.[3,4] Improved techniques of bowel preparation, antibiotics, alkalinizing agents and the development of newer absorbable suture materials further minimized the number of postoperative complications.

Once these problems had been solved, continence gained importance. In patients with ureterosigmoidostomy or a rectal bladder, frequency and urgency were often observed and high rates of night-time incontinence were reported.[5–7] Urodynamic investigations in bladder substitutes and rectal reservoirs showed that bowel contractions with a pressure rise in the reservoir are responsible for the incontinence.[5,8,9] By interrupting the circular contractions (antimesenteric opening of the bowel and 'reconfiguration'), a low-pressure reservoir is created, thus improving continence rates and protecting the upper urinary tract.[10]

The first attempt to lower the pressure in rectal reservoirs was made by Kock et al.,[9] who reported a method of urinary diversion to the rectum augmented by an ileal patch. This technique is elaborate and time-consuming. By antimesenteric opening of the rectosigmoid junction and simple side-to-side anastomosis, a low-pressure reservoir is equally created. This technique has been termed the sigma–rectum pouch (Mainz pouch II).[11,12]

Patients and methods

Surgical technique

At the junction between the sigmoid colon and rectum, the intestine is opened at the taenia libera over a length of 10–12 cm, both distal and proximal to this point. A pouch plate is created by side-to-side anastomosis of the medial margins by two-layer running sutures using 4/0 polyglyconate for the seromuscular layer and 4/0 catgut for the mucosa. The ureters are implanted lateral and parallel to the median running suture using the Goodwin–Hohenfellner technique through a submucosal tunnel (Fig. 17.1) and stented. The pouch is fixed to the anterior longitudinal cord of the promontory or to the psoas muscle to guarantee a straight ureteral path and avoid kinking. For closure of the anterior pouch wall, a two-layer running suture (mucosa and seromuscular) is used. The pouch is drained by a bowel tube for 3–4 days. The ureteral splints are removed at about day 8 after operation.

Patients

Between November 1990 and August 1993, the authors undertook this surgical procedure in 73 patients, including 14 children, at their institution. Patients' mean age was 43.5 years (range 10 months to 72

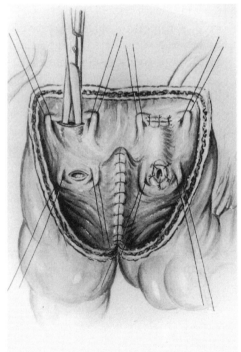

Figure 17.1. After antimesenteric opening of the bowel and side-to-side anastomosis of the medial margins the ureters are implanted parallel using the Goodwin–Hohenfellner technique.

years). The indications were malignancy in 55 patients, bladder exstrophy or incontinent epispadias in 14, traumatic loss of the urethra in two and a sinus urogenitalia with incontinence in one patient. Five early complications in four of the 73 patients (6.8%) were encountered: these were a dislodged ureteral stent, one pulmonary embolism, one case of pneumonia, one suture dehiscence and one ileus requiring operative intervention.

Results

In 69 patients the mean follow-up period was 12.7 months (range 1–30 months); the other four patients died of infiltrating cancer. Eight late complications required surgical intervention (11%): stenosis at the ureteral implantation site required reimplantation in five patients; there was one case of nephrolithiasis followed by extracorporal shock wave treatment; rupture of the anterior running suture line of the pouch necessitated a temporary colostomy and subsequent surgical revision in one patient, and one case of perianal bleeding under chemotherapy was treated by endoscopic coagulation. During follow-up, six patients presented with pyelonephritis (4.5% of renal units).

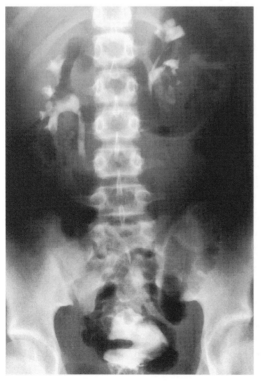

Figure 17.2. Postoperative intravenous urogram of a 12-year-old girl with bladder exstrophy after resection of the bladder plate and sigma–rectum pouch.

Of the 73 patients, 69 were completely continent postoperatively (daytime continence 94.5%) (Fig. 17.2). Four patients suffered from stress incontinence (grade I–II); one of these patients is also incontinent during the night (night-time continence 98.6%). Alkalinizing drugs are taken regularly by 49 patients to avoid metabolic acidosis. Hyperchloraemic acidosis has been observed in only two patients, who refused any alkalinizing medication.

Discussion

In 1969, in an attempt to construct a continent faecal reservoir, Kock[14] showed that a closed loop bowel segment, large or small, was capable of generating significant contractions. The rapid development of different forms of continent urinary diversion by creating reservoirs of various segments of the intestinal tract renewed interest in changes in motility after diversion procedures. It is clear that the overall goal in the construction of such reservoirs is the storage of large amounts of urine for a reasonable time under low pressure. The pressure in the intact sigmoid colon can reach up to 200 cmH_2O during defaecation and the pressure waves that reach the distal colon with mass movements are in the order of 60–80 cmH_2O. These high-pressure conditions within the sigmoid colon and rectum, caused by physiological bowel contractions, were regarded as major causes of recurrent pyelonephritis as well as of nocturnal incontinence. Consequently, all subsequent modifications of ureterosigmoidostomy were aimed at reducing pressure within the rectosigmoid.

Ghoneim, initially having used a modification of the Mauclaire procedure,[13,14] decided to augment the rectosigmoid with a segment of ileum, thus creating the so-called 'augmented rectal bladder'.[15] As oral administration of alkalinizing drugs is problematic, because of poor patient compliance and limited possibilities of follow-up, the development of acidosis had to be prevented by other means. Urine could reflux into the descending and transverse colon and the large absorbent surface would increase the risk of biochemical disruption. For this reason, a valve mechanism was placed above the ileal patch in order to prevent urine ascending into high bowel segments. The valve mechanism was created from sigmoid colon, which was invaginated and fixed by staples. A temporary colostomy, which was closed after 6–8 weeks, was placed for protection.

This technique, however, had several distinct disadvantages. A bowel anastomosis had to be performed in order to use the ileal patch; staples had to be used to secure the bowel invagination; last but not least, a second operative intervention was necessary in order to close the colostomy. All these additional steps are fraught with complications and have converted the simple technique of ureterosigmoidostomy into an elaborate and complex procedure.

By applying Hinman's principles of intestinal detubularization, the present authors have developed a novel modification of the classical technique of ureterosigmoidostomy, the sigma–rectum pouch (Mainz pouch II).[12] The idea was to lower the pressure within the rectosigmoid, not by an elaborate augmentation but by simple detubularization, leaving the bowel in continuity. Detubularization of the intestinal tract eliminates mass contractions and high-pressure peaks. In addition, the theoretical volume of the reservoir is increased.[10,16,17]

The annals of surgical literature reveal that so-called 'state-of-the-art' concepts, which are believed to have developed from years of sophisticated clinical and basic scientific research, are really not novel. Often, if the time is taken to study 'ancient' literature, many current concepts are found to have been proposed previously, but for some reason were not accepted at that time. For example, back in 1907 Kocher[18] proposed a most beneficial modification of the Maydl procedure (implantation of the trigone into the sigmoid colon) by means of distal sigmoid–sigmoid side-to-side anastomosis and he did so without the advanced knowledge of bowel motility and pressure conditions. However, in 1903 the time for detubularization had not yet come and his idea was forgotten. A similar example is Goodwin's technique for ureterosigmoidostomy. The literature does not pay adequate tribute to this modification. His open (trans-sigmoid) ureteral implantation not only had the advantage of a more technically simpler implantation, owing to better exposure, but also, and more important, by means of the longitudinal antimesenteric incision of the sigmoid and subsequent two-layer closure, the tight mucosa-to-mucosa suture and the relaxed seromuscular suture, a form of myotomy was performed. Daniels subsequently compared Goodwin's technique with other, similar, modifications and confirmed the establishment of a lower pressure within the sigmoid on using Goodwin's technique.[19]

During the past century the original surgical technique for internal urinary diversion[1] has been varied in many respects. Since the often-cited publication by Simon in 1852 more than 60 modifications of ureterosigmoidostomy have been published.[2] In the long term, many of them appeared only to make matters worse. Critics of ureterosigmoidostomy still tend to cite publications dealing with complications of ureterosigmoidostomy in patients operated on before the 1950s,[20] a time at which many problems relating to this technique were still unsolved, owing to lack of the above-mentioned materials and drugs. Ironically, the proclamation that ureterosigmoidostomy should probably be abandoned[21] coincided with the triumph of the ileal conduit.[22] Several series are currently demonstrating a low rate of early complications and acceptable long-term results using ureterosigmoidostomy, and seem to herald a type of renaissance of this surgical technique. Unfavourable long-term results of ileal conduit diversions support this trend.[23–29]

Although ureterosigmoidostomy is associated with complications, as are most forms of urinary diversion, the knowledge of these potential problems through over a century of application permits many such complications to be anticipated and treated before they become serious medical problems. In correctly selected patients requiring a continent urinary diversion, and with close monitoring (which has to be performed after any form of urinary diversion), ureterosigmoidostomy represents a viable alternative to other surgical techniques.

After 25 years of experience of classical ureterosigmoidostomy in well over 300 cases, the authors consider that the sigma–rectum pouch has many other advantages over other forms of continent urinary diversion. A reservoir capacity (200–300 ml), the safe and stable pouch fixation in the area of the promontory guaranteeing a straight ureteral path, as well as the low pressure even at high filling volumes, make the sigma–rectum pouch a most attractive alternative to many forms of continent urinary diversion. The surgical technique described, termed the Mainz pouch II, may help to obviate or minimize the traditional deficiencies of classical ureterosigmoidostomy and may lead to a renaissance of that procedure.

References

1. Simon J. Extropia vesicae (absence of the anterior walls of the bladder and pubic abdominal parieties): operation for directing the orifices of the ureters into the rectum; temporary success; subsequent death; autopsy. Lancet 1852; 2: 568–569
2. Hinman F, Weyrauch H M Jr. A critical study of the different principles of surgery which have been used in uretero–intestinal implantation. Trans Am Assoc Genito-Urin Surg 1936; 29: 15
3. Leadbetter W F. Considerations of problems incident to performance of ureterenterostomy. J Urol 1951; 65: 818
4. Goodwin W E, Harris A P, Kaufman J J, Beal J M. Open, transcolonic ureterointestinal anastomosis: a new approach. Surg Gynecol Obstet 1953; 97: 295
5. Ghoneim M A, Shebab-El-Din A B, Ashamallah A K, Gaballah M A. Evolution of the rectal bladder as a method for urinary diversion. J Urol 1981; 126: 737
6. McConnel J B, Stewart W K. The long-term management and social consequences of ureterosigmoid anastomosis. Br J Urol 1975; 47: 607
7. Boyce W H. A new concept concerning treatment of exstrophy of the bladder: 20 years later. J Urol 1972; 107: 476
8. Leisinger H J, Säuberli H, Schauwecker H, Mayor G. Continent ileal bladder. Eur Urol 1976; 2: 8

9. Kock N G, Ghoneim M A, Lycke K G, Mahrab M R. Urinary diversion to the augmented and valved rectum: preliminary results with a novel surgical procedure. J Urol 1988; 140: 1375

10. Hinman F Jr. Selection of intestinal segments for bladder substitution: physical and physiological characteristics. J Urol 1988; 139: 519

11. Fisch M, Hohenfellner R. Der Sigma–Rektum Pouch: Eine Modifikation der Harnleiterdarmimplantation. Aktuel Urol 1991; 22: 1

12. Fisch M, Wammack R, Müller S C, Hohenfellner R. The Mainz Pouch II (Sigma Rectum Pouch). J Urol 1993; 149: 258

13. Hohenfellner R, Wulff H D. Zur Harnableitung mittels ausgeschalteter Dickdarmsegmente. Aktuel Urol 1970; 1: 18

14. Kock N G. Intra-abdominal 'reservoir' in patients with permanent ileostomy. Preliminary observations on a procedure resulting in fecal 'continence' in five ileostomy patients. Arch Surg 1969; 99: 223

15. Ghoneim M A, Shoukry I. The rectal bladder with perineal colostomy for urinary diversion. Urology 1974; 4: 511

16. Koff S A. Guidelines to determine the size and shape of intestinal segments used for reconstruction. J Urol 1988; 140: 1150

17. Hohenfellner R, Planz C, Wulff H D et al. Die transsigmoidale Ureterostomie (Sigma–Rektum Blase): Operationstechnik und Gesamtkörperkaliumbestimmung. Urologe 1967; 6: 275

18. Kocher T. Chirurgische Operationslehre. Jena: Gustav Fischer, 1907: 1017

19. Connor J P, Hensle T W, Lattimer J K, Burbige K A. Long-term followup of 207 patients with bladder exstrophy: an evolution in treatment. J Urol 1989; 142: 793

20. Stamey T A. The pathogenesis and implications of the electrolyte imbalance in ureterosigmoidostomy. Surg Gynecol Obstet 1956; 103: 736

21. Bricker E M. Bladder substitution after pelvic evisceration. Surg Clin North Am 1950; 30: 1511

22. Schwarz G R, Jeffs R D. Ileal conduit urinary diversion in children: computer analysis of follow-up from 2–16 years. J Urol 1975; 114: 285

23. Shapiro S R, Lebowitz R, Colodny A H. Fate of 90 children with ileal conduit diversion a decade later: analysis of complications, pyelography, renal function and bacteriology. J Urol 1975; 114: 289

24. Middleton A W, Hendren W H. Ileal conduits in children at the Massachusetts General Hospital from 1955 to 1970. J Urol 1976; 115: 591

25. Johnson D E, Lamy S M. Complications of a single stage radical cystectomy and ileal conduit diversion: review of 214 cases. J Urol 1977; 117: 171

26. Mitchell M E, Yoder I C, Pfister R C. Ileal loop stenosis: a late complication of urinary diversion. J Urol 1977; 118: 957

27. Sullivan J W, Grabstald H, Whitmore W F Jr. Complications of ureteroileal conduit with radical cystectomy: review of 336 cases. J Urol 1980; 124: 797

28. Kamidono S, Oda Y, Hamami G et al. Urinary diversion: anastomosis of the ureters into a sigmoid pouch and end-to-side sigmoidorectostomy. J Urol 1985; 133: 391

29. Hendren W H, Radopoulos D. Complications of ileal loop and colon conduit urinary diversion. Urol Clin North Am 1983; 10: 451

18

Congenital neuropathic bladder: concepts, indications and pitfalls of reconstructive surgery

E. J. McGuire

Background

The congenital neuropathic bladder generally implies conditions associated with myelodysplasia, and/or sacral agenesis. Cerebral palsy is associated on occasion with neurogenic vesical dysfunction, but this rarely calls for reconstruction.

The most striking feature of the congenital neuropathic bladder, beyond the risk of development of upper tract disease, is the prevalence of incontinence. That problem is due to the general character of the condition and is not related to the age of the patient population. The great challenge in these patients is to restore continence without jeopardizing upper tract function.[1]

Development

Most children with myelodysplasia or sacral agenesis demonstrate at birth an areflexic bladder with an open, non-functional urethra from the vesical outlet to the pelvic floor.[2] If any urethral closure in these patients is preserved — and in almost every instance there is some urethral closure — it is manifested in the area of the pelvic diaphragm or more precisely, extrinsic part of the striated sphincter innervated by the pudendal nerve[3] (Fig. 18.1).

A smaller number of children, 5–6%, are born with a normal lower urinary tract, including normal reflex function of the bladder with coordinate behaviour of the sphincters. At rest, the vesical outlet is closed and the internal sphincter provides adequate continence function.[4]

About 10–20% of these children show a reflex bladder with a closed internal sphincter at rest and reflexly determined detrusor external

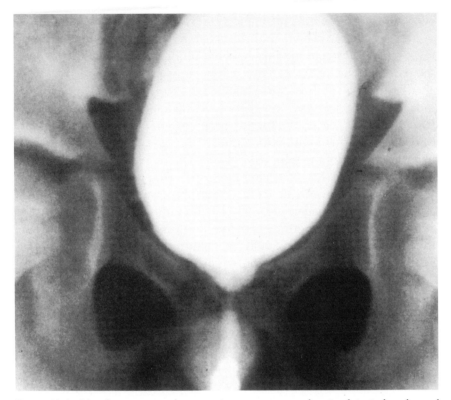

Figure 18.1. Upright cystogram demonstrating an open non-functional vesical outlet and proximal urethra to the mid-urethral level. Study is of a 4-year-old myelodysplastic girl.

sphincter dyssynergia identical to that seen in spinal cord injury patients with transverse upper motor neuron lesions, and functional sacral cord segments distal to the transverse lesion.[2–4]

Given the nature and extent of the cord abnormalities described in patients with myelodysplasia and sacral agenesis, it is not surprising that a lower motor neuron type picture is more common than an upper motor neuron lesion associated with detrusor sphincter dyssynergia. The latter condition requires a functioning cord distal to the lesion. As a general rule, the higher the lesion in a meningomyelocoele patient, the less likely is the presence of a congenital neuropathic bladder, despite other abnormalities.

Neurosurgical procedures and function of the lower urinary tract

The initial neurosurgical treatment, including closure of the neural and meningeal defect, as well as the cutaneous defect, and ventricular peritoneal shunting for communicating hydrocephalus, generally results in little substantial change in the expression of the neurogenic bladder in these children, except for a decrease in sphincter pressure recorded from the extrinsic part of the external sphincter or pelvic diaphragm.[2,5] That change reduces, at least for a time, the detrusor pressure required to induce urinary leakage. In addition, temporary large-volume urinary retention may occur following back closure, which may require intermittent catheterization for a time or, in some cases, has been treated by hyperdilation of the sphincter.[6–8]

During the first few years after birth, including the period until school age, the primary treatment effort is directed toward preservation of low pressures in the bladder, generally by intermittent catheterization and occasionally by intermittent catheterization and drugs. In cases where the bladder pressure cannot be controlled by these measures, vesicostomy, or sphincter dilation, can be used.[2,4,5]

When school age is attained, or serious problems with bladder storage function occur alone or in conjunction with upper tract abnormalities, reconstruction of the urinary tract becomes important for social reasons relating to continence, as well as to prevent renal or ureteral damage.[9] In some cases, unfortunately, renal damage may be so severe, related to neuropathic dysfunction, that reconstructive surgery is only a prerequisite to renal transplantation.[10]

Assessment of urinary tract status before reconstruction

Patients may present with an intact but poorly functional urinary tract, or one already changed by previous surgery and no longer in continuity.

Intact urinary systems
Assessment must provide basic data on renal, ureteral, bladder and urethral function.

Ureteral function
The basic requirement is for ureteral peristalsis. Ureteral size or appearance are not as important as peristalsis. In an intact system, ureteral work is defined and determined by intravesical storage pressures or bladder 'compliance'. When the bladder requires reconstruction, or when a neo-reservoir is to be constructed because the bladder is missing or so badly damaged as to be abandoned, the ureter can be examined during urine formation and flow with reservoir factors *obviated*: that is, the bladder can be emptied continuously during a renogram, or ultrasound assessment of ureteral peristalsis, or during a Whitaker perfusion test.

If, on the other hand, the bladder is felt to be adequate for low-pressure storage, ureteral function should be judged against various incremental pressures and volumes known to be achieved by *that* bladder. Inspection of bladder pressure–volume curves is essential before testing for ureteral function if the bladder is to be left intact, and not reconstructed (Fig. 18.2a, b).

In young children, some with dilated large ureters, Weiss found that ureteral peristalsis visible on ultrasound was sufficient evidence for ureteral function to proceed with reconstruction.[11] In older children, the value of that finding has not been established, although Pohl found ureteral size to be independent of force generation within the ureter when measured experimentally.[12] That would suggest that a wide ureter is not necessarily a bad ureter, and vice versa.

If there is doubt about ureteral competence, a perfusion test, under fluoroscopic monitoring, provides the best overall information or ureteral function. If that study shows low-pressure fluid transfer into the bladder, or elsewhere, or through the terminus of the ureter, without difficulty, or undue pressure, the ureter is capable of fluid transfer into a low-pressure reservoir (Fig. 18.3).

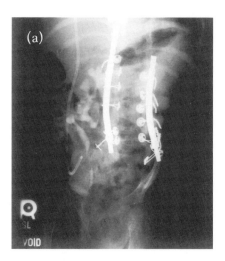 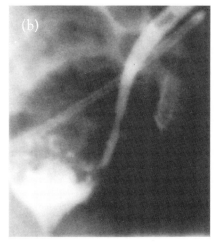

Figure 18.2. (a) Intravenous urogram from an infant girl with myelodysplasia treated for bilateral grade 4 vesicoureteral reflux, by bilateral loop cutaneous ureterostomies. Note ventriculoperitoneal shunt, and reasonable decompression of the upper tracts and ureters, which were massively dilated. (b) Same child as in (a), at the age of 2 years. Note the open bladder outlet. Whitaker perfusion testing via the cutaneous ureterostomy was normal with the bladder emptied continuously by a Foley catheter. At 30 ml bladder volume, detrusor pressure rose to 48 cmH$_2$O and the Whitaker perfusion test became very high pressure positive.

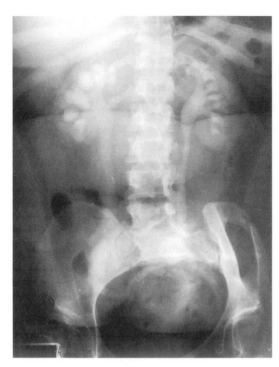

Figure 18.3. Intravenous urogram from a 6-year-old child with myelodysplasia showing bilateral hydroureter, at a large bladder volume. Visible vigorous ureteral peristalsis was present on stereoscopic observation. Despite the size, the ureteral function can be assumed to be satisfactory if a low-pressure reservoir is achieved.

Bladder function and urethral function

In congenital neuropathic conditions, the presence or absence of reflex vesical contractility should be documented. In addition, a very careful assessment of bladder compliance, or the ability of the bladder to store urine at low pressure, is critical. Those children or adults with sacral agenesis or myelodysplasia who can be demonstrated to have a reflex bladder contraction will also demonstrate a normally closed internal sphincter mechanism. Individuals with areflex bladder dysfunction will, almost invariably, lack closure of the internal sphincter mechanism. In the former situation — a reflex bladder with or without detrusor sphincter dyssynergia — the internal sphincter mechanism will be an effective organ of resistance to abdominal pressure as an expulsive force: the normally closed internal sphincter will not leak with effort, transfers, coughing, and/or other vigorous activity. For purposes of reconstruction, a normally closed urethra, or one closed at the bladder neck, which opens only with a reflex contraction, need not be changed in any way, before or at the time of reconstruction.

Children with myelodysplasia who exhibit reflex detrusor sphincter dyssynergia will almost always demonstrate high to very high intravesical pressures; for that reason, many will have undergone urinary diversion early in their life, or will have been subjected to vesicostomy. Bloom and coworkers showed that children with detrusor sphincter dyssynergia, if identified at an early stage by the presence of high detrusor pressures at the time of voiding and treated by intermittent catheterization and drugs, were quite often rendered completely continent and preserved normal bladder compliance indefinitely.[3,13]

Urethral functional assessment The most useful method for evaluation of sphincter function is measurement of the abdominal pressure component of the total bladder pressure that induces leakages. That can be done with the subject upright, or nearly so, and the bladder filled to approximately one-half capacity, by inducing an increase in abdominal pressure with straining until a pressure of 150 cmH_2O is reached or leakage occurs.[14] A urethra that tolerates an abdominal pressure of 150 cmH_2O without leakage is either normal or will resist abdominal pressure sufficiently well to render unnecessary a separate procedure on the urethra. In measuring the abdominal pressure to cause leakage, it is important to be sure that the detrusor pressure component with filling is minimal, at least to the volume attained at the time the test is done. If compliance is poor, the proximal urethra becomes progressively incorporated into the bladder as bladder pressure rises. In that case (and often, after prolonged bladder defunctionalization, bladder compliance is very poor) it may be impossible to ascertain whether the urethra is open because it does not work, or is forced open by an increase in intravesical pressure.

Bladder factors If reflex, uncontrolled, vesical activity is present but can be suppressed using drugs and there is no abnormality of compliance (which situation after the age of 2 or 3 years would be unusual or unlikely) the bladder can be judged 'normal' enough to need no further treatment apart from the institution of intermittent catheterization.

If reflex activity is present but compliance is poor, outlet ablative procedures such as vesicostomy or sphincterotomy may induce lower intravesical pressure and restore compliance to some extent, but these are not useful because of their effect on continence. Such procedures, although effectively minimizing the risk of upper tract damage and preserving upper tract integrity, are not 'reconstructive'.

If compliance is poor in association with an areflex bladder (which has not been defunctionalized), some procedure that will produce a large low-pressure reservoir is generally required. Cyclic filling and other distension techniques have not been very useful in patients with congenital neuropathic vesical dysfunction associated with poor compliance.[15]

Vesicoureteral reflux

The presence of vesicoureteral reflux complicates assessment of the intact lower urinary tract because, when present, it precludes determination of an accurate pressure–volume curve from the bladder. Although primary reflux does occur in this patient group, the more usual cause is elevated intravesical pressure. When intravesical pressure is dissipated by vesicoureteral reflux, in effect part of the reservoir function of the bladder becomes the compliance of the ureters, which is an unhealthy situation. Video monitoring during bladder pressure–volume testing is essential in this patient population to identify vesicoureteral reflux and thus to assess a falsely negative cystometrogram or pressure–volume curve.

If vesicoureteral reflux occurs, it is often worse on one side than the other. That finding does not imply primary reflux due to 'valvular' dysfunction. If the detrusor pressure required to cause leakage is 40 cmH$_2$O or more, produced either by reflex or areflex bladder contractility vesicoureteral reflux can be presumed to be pressure related.

In children with exstrophy who are evaluated for reconstruction, primary valvular failure, perhaps due to maldevelopment of the trigone, is common, and persistent vesicoureteral reflux may be seen even in association with very large low-pressure reservoirs constructed from various bowel segments.

In children or adults with reflux, but active, ureteral peristalsis and relatively normal size ureters, it is not usually necessary to reimplant the ureters as part of the reconstruction procedure, provided that a low-pressure reservoir is attained.[15] This presupposes a definitive diagnosis of poor compliance and/or high leak-point pressures in association with vesicoureteral reflux.

Discontinuous urinary systems

Supravesical diversion hinders assessment of bladder reservoir function. Unlike renal transplantation candidates in renal failure for non-urological reasons, patients treated by ileal loop diversion or cutaneous ureterostomy for congenital neuropathic bladder disease will not reliably regain comfortable bladder function without a major reconstruction. A defunctionalized bladder following supravesical diversion can be assumed to be physically small and to have little or no potential to expand spontaneously. Augmentation cystoplasty or neoreservoir construction may be undertaken, discarding the bladder and the urethra.[15,16] When a neuropathic bladder and urethra are left behind, pyocystitis and continued problems with fluid leakage, infection and pain are common. If the bladder is present, the author usually incorporates it into the reconstruction, to prevent the development of pyocystits, and to avoid the necessity for cystectomy.

Catheterization

The ability to catheterize the native urethra, or a neourethral segment constructed of bowel of bladder, is often essential to overall outcome. Patient motivation is also an important aspect in overall outcome, particularly in teenagers, where failure to carry out intermittent catheterization may be a problem.

Renal function

Normal creatinine clearance is not a prerequisite for reconstructive surgery. Ureteral peristalsis is an absolute requirement, but renal damage by pyelonephritis, the presence of upper tract stones, and/or diminished renal function are frequently stabilized or halted by achievement of a closed system where the ureters drain into a low-pressure reservoir emptied by intermittent catheterization.[15]

Basic goals

The ultimate goal is the creation of a urinary system that permits a normal life. To achieve that, a closed upper tract system with a low-pressure accumulation reservoir and a competent valve for continence are required. Although the reservoir can safely be emptied periodically by catheterization, or by other means, there is no way to replace low-pressure storage in any continent system. Reservoir compliance, or volume tolerance, is an absolute requirement for any reconstructive procedure.

Conservative measures

It is now clear that both neurogenic and obstructive conditions that produce a situation in which the detrusor muscle interacts with abnormal outlet resistance can induce a dramatic change in detrusor muscular behaviour, and ultimately can produce changes in the viscoelastic properties of the bladder wall itself.[13] The end result of these processes, triggered by detrusor–outlet interaction, is loss of reservoir function due to fibrosis. At an early stage the primary muscular changes may be completely reversible, especially in younger individuals where the process of detrusor–outlet interaction has not been prolonged.

Bloom and coworkers[5] have shown that poor compliance in myelodysplastic children can often be prevented by the early imposition of intermittent catheterization and, if necessary, anticholinergic agents. The treatments often prevented the development of poor compliance, or resulted in improvement of compliance that was already abnormal. If either treatment was ineffective or was started too late, transient outlet pressure reduction achieved by dilation of the urethra resulted in a dramatic change in compliance in the children in question.[13] Similar findings have been reported in patients with spinal cord injury who were started on intermittent catheterization programmes at a very early stage.[17]

If these conservative measures fail and compliance remains poor, some treatment is mandatory to preserve urethral and renal function. Generally, that treatment is directed at achievement of a large low-pressure reservoir, although sphincter ablative procedures on the outlet have a similar effect.

Procedures to improve reservoir function

Partial excision of the detrusor musculature

Detrusor muscular excision is a relatively new development but detrusor muscle incisions have been used previously in enuretic children with limited success. Snow and Cartwright recently described a technique in which the detrusor muscle is carefully removed from the underlying bladder mucosa and lamina propria and discarded.[18] The original authors intended to create a pressure-relieving diverticulum-like structure. Other workers have excised more of the detrusor, in fact as much of the detrusor muscle is feasible, taking the superior vesical pedicles on both sides, and removing the detrusor from the anterior, lateral and superior surfaces of the bladder mucosa[19] (Fig. 18.4a–c). Inadvertent mucosal injuries are closed with small absorbable sutures. Absolute removal of all muscle is not required.

The combined experience at the University of Michigan, the University of Texas and that reported by Stöhrer in Murnau, Germany, involves 54 patients. Results, with respect to good reservoir function, are excellent in 75% or more. Failure may be related to gross extravasation with subsequent fibrosis over the superior surface of the bladder. The long-term outcome after myomectomy is not yet known.[18,19]

Augmentation cystoplasty

When compliance is poor, or when the bladder is physically small owing to long-term defunctionalization, or when a long-term vesicostomy makes myomectomy impossible, augmentation cystoplasty is an excellent alternative to supravesical diversion or continent total diversion.

Augmentation cystoplasty preserves the trigone and the bladder, which prevents the development of pyocystitis and avoids the necessity for cystectomy. It is easier than a full continent diversion and the results

(a)

(b)

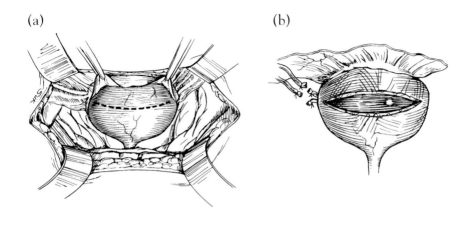

(c)

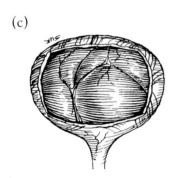

Figure 18.4. Detrusor myomectomy: (a) incision line in the detrusor muscle carried down to the mucosal surface made with a 15 blade; (b) mobilization of the peritoneum is complete, and excision of the detrusor muscle from the underlying mucosa is underway; (c) completed procedure. The detrusor muscle has been excised from the mucosal surface as completely as is feasible. Small remnants of muscle fibres remain, which is a perfectly acceptable situation.

are predictable. The author's usual choice is to construct a reservoir from small bowel which is detubularized and sutured to the bladder in the manner depicted in Fig. 18.5a–f. This procedure necessitates intermittent catheterization, and children who are undiverted into such reservoirs must be watched to be certain they are compliant with the intermittent catheterization protocol. Frequent intermittent catheterization is initiated on or about postoperative day 7, with integrity of the reservoir confirmed by fluoroscopic cystography. The function of each reservoir is monitored with pressure–volume curves every 3 months, and endoscopy at 6-monthly intervals. Metal staples, which are associated with stone formation, should be avoided in any of these procedures.

In a series reported by the author, 120 patients were treated by augmentation cystoplasty and followed for at least 6 months with a mean of 37 months, and a range from 6 to 96 months. The following findings were noted. Bladder capacity, defined as bladder volume at a pressure of 38 cmH$_2$O, increased from a mean preoperative value of 108 ml to

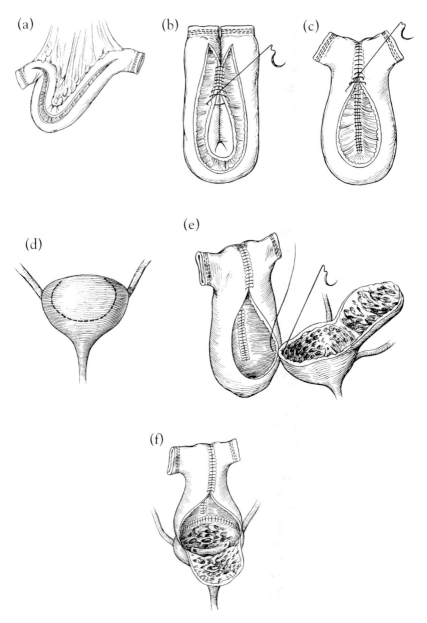

Figure 18.5. Augmentation cystoplasty: (a) a small bowel segment (18–24 cm) is selected, and incised along its antimesenteric border; (b) the posterior wall of the 'neoreservoir' is closed with a running suture of absorbable material; (c) partial closure of the anterior wall of the neoreservoir leaves a large open inferior segment involving the lower half of the pouch; (d) the incision line in the bladder creates an anteriorly based large detrusor flap; (e) the anastomosis of the bowel segment to the open bladder is depicted; the posterior/inferior suture line is placed first through the lumen of the neoreservoir; (f) completed posterior/lateral suture lines. The anterior closure fits the bladder flap into the open reservoir.

438 ml with a range of 200–1200 ml postoperatively. There was a dramatic effect on compliance and upper tract function was preserved, stabilized or improved. However, five patients developed small bowel obstruction, two requiring surgical intervention for this problem; 22% developed reservoir calculi; five patients developed apparent reservoir rupture, three requiring open operative drainage and repair, but the other two resolving their problem with conservative therapy comprising mainly intravenous fluids, antimicrobials and bed rest.

Procedures on the urethra

A urethra that leaks urine, may be incompetent, but it must be determined whether the urinary leakage is due to lack of resistance to reservoir (detrusor) pressure or to abdominal pressure, as these are not identical forces. Generally, lack of resistance to reservoir pressure requires treatment of the reservoir rather than of the urethra. In some cases urethral function is so poor that it is better to construct a neourethra from the appendix or ileum and to close the native urethra.[16]

When a urethra is constructed or reconstructed in a manner that ensures continence by a compressive effect exerted by detrusor pressure on the 'urethra' as, for example, in the Mitrofanoff technique, or the Kropp urethral reimplantation, augmentation of the bladder by some measure is *mandatory*. The infinite resistance offered by these surgically constructed 'urethras' will engender a pressure response in the detrusor, which results in loss of compliance and a clear risk to upper tract function.

The urethral sphincter can be assumed to be adequate (against bladder pressure) if it resists detrusor pressure to 20 cmH$_2$O. That can be assessed by bladder leak-point pressure measurement or, in the case of those with meningomyelocoeles or sacral agenesis, by measurement of maximum urethral pressure (UPP), provided that the bladder is areflexic. The maximum UPP value will reflect resistance to detrusor pressure. If the bladder leak-point pressure or the maximum urethral closing pressure are high, 30 cmH$_2$O or more, if must be ascertained whether the bladder is storing urine normally; if not, this must be assured surgically.

Resistance of the urethral sphincter to abdominal pressure is an entirely different matter. That function is unrelated to pressure in the urethra, particularly UPP. It is measurable by determination of the abdominal pressure required to induce leakage. In individuals with a meningomyelocele or sacral agenesis, an open non-functional sphincter is easy to diagnose on upright cystography (see Fig. 18.1). The internal sphincter can be closed by a sling procedure, by collagen injection, or by an artificial sphincter.[20,21] Collagen and slings change intrinsic urethral

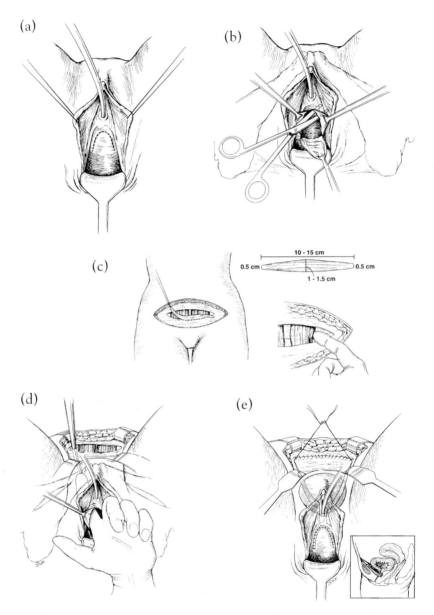

(a)

(b)

(c)

10 - 15 cm

0.5 cm   0.5 cm

1 - 1.5 cm

(d)

(e)

Figure 18.6. Pubovaginal sling: (a) the vaginal incision; (b) entry to the retropubic space is made sharply, lateral to the urethra, immediately adjacent to the ischium; (c) excision of the sling from the interior leaf of rectus abdominis fascia to expose the entry point into the retropubic space from above; that point is just lateral to the insertion of the rectus abdominis muscle on the pubic symphysis where there is a defect in the fascial closure of the abdominal wall; (d) creation of a passage for the sling under bimanual control; (e) sling sutures are tied over the rectus fascia almost to occlude the vesical outlet. Sling tension need not be excessive, and finger or clamp should slide easily under the tied sling sutures between the sutures and the rectus abdominis fascia.

closing pressure only very slightly and do not influence the bladder leak-point pressure. The artificial sphincter is nearly as effective against detrusor pressure as it is against abdominal pressure and thus, has a potential effect on compliance. Overall results with slings in female patients are excellent, with 80–95% dry on long-term follow-up.[20] The procedure is relatively easy, even in young children, and requires only about 40 min operating time (Fig. 18.6a–e). Long-term results with collagen are not yet available but early results indicate good to very good results in female patients with neuropathic vesical dysfunction but less satisfactory results in male patients (Fig. 18.7a, b). The artificial sphincter remains the best method to ensure continence in males at present, although slings can also be used. Careful follow-up is required after implantation of a sphincter, to prevent the late effects of that procedure on bladder compliance.

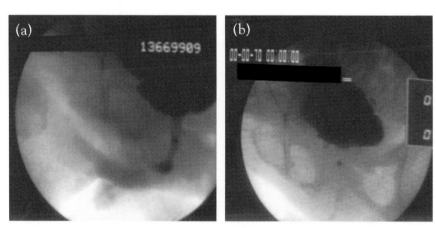

Figure 18.7. (a) Upright cystogram from a male patient with myelodysplasia showing egress of contrast at very low abnormal pressure (13 cmH$_2$O – detrusor component) across the sphincter manifesting a pressure of 33 cmH$_2$O. (b) Same patient after collagen injection, showing resistance of the internal sphincter to an abdominal pressure of 54 cmH$_2$O.

References

1. Steinburg M, Bennett C, Konnak J et al. Construction of a low pressure reservoir and achievement of continence after diversion and in end stage vesical dysfunction. J Urol 1987; 138: 39

2. Wang S C, McGuire E J, Bloom D A. A bladder pressure management system for myelodysplasia — clinical outcome. J Urol 1988; 140: 1459

3. McGuire E J, Woodside J R, Borden T A, Weiss R M. Prognostic value of urodynamic testing in myelodysplastic patients. J Urol 1981; 126: 205

4. McGuire E J. Mielodisplasia: pathophysiologie, neuroanatomia, correlata e manifestazioni urologiche. J Pediatr Neurosci 1985; 1: 4

5. Bloom D A, McGuire E J. Practical management of children with myelomeningecele. In: Ehrlich R M (ed) Dialogues in pediatric urology. New York: Miller, 1989; 12(6): 3–4

6. Johnson J H, Farkas A. Congenital neurogenic bladder: practicalities and possiblities of conservative management. Urology 1975; 5: 719

7. Johnson J R, Kathel B L. The obstructed neurogenic bladder in the new born. Br J Urol 1971; 43: 206

8. Shochat S J, Perlmutter A D. Myelodysplasia neonatal hydronephrosis: the value of urethral dilation. J Urol 1972; 107: 146

9. Ghoneim G M, Bloom D A, McGuire E J, Stewart K L. Bladder compliance in meningomyelocele children. J Urol 1989; 14: 1404

10. Zaragoza M R, Ritchey M L, Bloom D A et al. Cystoplasty in renal transplantation candidates: urodynamic evaluation and outcome. J Urol 1993; 150: 1463

11. Weiss R M. The implications of the dilated upper urinary tract: diagnostic dilemmas. In: Lytton B (ed) Advances in urology. Chicago: Year Book Medical, 1988; 1: 1

12. Pohl J, Dambacher J, Sulke J, Holzknecht A. In vivo measurement of force in the urethra. Urology Int 1991; 46: 313

13. Bloom D A, Knechtel J M, McGuire E J. Urethral dilation improves bladder compliance in children with myelomeningocele and high leak point pressures. J Urol 1990; 144: 430

14. McGuire E J, Fitzpatrick C C, Wan J et al. Clinical assessment of urethral sphincter function. J Urol 1993; 150: 1452

15. Key D, Wan J, Grainger R et al. Urinary tract reconstruction: applied urodynamics. Neurourol Urodyn 1990; 9: 509

16. Wan J, McGuire E J. Cystoplasty and closure of the urethra for the destroyed lower urinary tract. J Am Paraplegia Soc 1990; 13: 40

17. McGuire E J, Noll F, Maynard F. A pressure management system for the neurogenic bladder after spinal cord injury. Neuroural Urodyn 1991; 10: 223

18. Snow B W, Cartwright P C. Autoaugmentation of the bladder. Contemp Urol 1992; 4: 41

19. Kennelly M J, Gormley E A, McGuire E J. Early clinical experience with adult bladder autoaugmentation. J Urol 1995; in press

20. Stöhrer M. Myomectomy in the treatment of neurogenic vesical dysfunction. Read at the Urodynamics Society Meeting, San Francisco, California, May 1994

21. Norbeck J C, McGuire E J. The use of pubovaginal and puboprostatic slings. Dialogues Ped Urol 1991; 14: 2

Maximal electrical stimulation for recurrent lower urinary tract infections and unstable bladder in children

19

B. Tršinar   M. Kralj

Introduction

In addition to micturition problems, such as enuresis, diurnal incontinence, urinary frequency and urgency, 45–70% of children with unstable bladder have recurrent infections of the lower urinary tract (UTI),[1-3] and 25–90% have vesicoureteral reflux (VUR).[4-6]

Mehrotra,[7] Finkbeiner and Lapides[8] and Siroky et al.[9] have proved by their experimental work that a temporarily or permanently increased infravesical pressure causes a 25–50% decrease in blood circulation in the bladder wall. This leads to a diminished production of the mucopolysaccharide (mucin) in the bladder mucosa that normally prevents adhesion of bacteria to the bladder cell membranes.[10] Binding of bacteria with their fimbriae to specific receptors of the bladder cells is the first condition for the development of UTI.

Increased intravesical pressure due to unstable bladder may be one of the factors responsible for the development of UTI.[2] Treatment of uninhibited detrusor contractions can be of great value in the sterilization of urine.[11,12]

A variety of more or less effective therapeutic modalities are available for the treatment of unstable bladder. These include drug therapy (oxybutinin, propantheline, terodiline),[13-15] special bladder training,[16] biofeedback therapy,[17,18] transvesical phenol injection,[19] bladder distension,[20] bladder transection[21] and acupuncture.[22]

Electrical stimulation (ES) of the lower urinary tract has also been recognized as an effective method for treating unstable bladder.[23-25] One of the available ES modalities, maximal electrical stimulation (MES), involves non-implantable short-term stimulation of the pelvic floor and has been used at the Department of Urology, University Medical Centre, Ljubljana, for 20 years. It employs vaginal or anal electrodes for stimulation of the afferent pudendal nerves, which, through the pudendal–pelvic spinal reflex, induces acute inhibition of unstable bladder.[26–28] The inhibitory effects of ES can be achieved by using electrical current of a relatively low intensity. The stimulating electrodes are placed close to the pudendal nerve, causing depolarization of the afferent pudendal fibres.[29,30] The so-called 'carry-over' therapeutic effect of periodic ES of the lower urinary tract is poorly understood. It may be due to the decreased activity or lower concentration of cholinergic receptors in the detrusor, or may occur as a result of reactivation of the 'lost' functional units.[31,32]

The aim of the study described in this chapter was to investigate the clinical and urodynamic effects of anal MES in children with recurrent UTI and unstable bladder.

Patients and methods

Treatment by MES was given to 39 girls, aged 5–17 years, mean age 9.7 years, with recurrent episodes of UTI, cystometrically proved detrusor instability and at least three positive urine cultures prior to the institution of therapy. *Escherichia coli* was isolated from 90% of the patients.

UTI at the time of urodynamic evaluation and MES was ruled out on the grounds of historical, clinical and laboratory data. Patients with neurogenic bladder, intravesical obstruction and organic bladder disease (e.g. fibrosis, calculi, papillomas) were excluded from the study. The diagnosis was established by ultrasound, micturition cystography and cystoscopy. Chronic cystitis was diagnosed in 13 girls and severe trabeculation of the detrusor in nine; in 18 patients 22 VURs were established.

The girls used a battery-powered electrical stimulator connected by a cable to the bipolar and plug electrodes (Fig. 19.1). The stimulator generated monophasic square current pulses with a duration of 1 ms and frequency of 20 Hz. After the plug electrode had been inserted into the anus, stimulation intensity was gradually increased up to the level of tolerable discomfort. MES was applied for 20 min daily for 1 month. After the termination of therapy, 36 children (three failed to attend for the follow-up) were followed up for 1–36 months (mean 12.4 months). They checked their own urine cultures every month. All patients received urinary antiseptics.

One month after the end of MES the girls were re-evaluated by water cystometry. The methods, definitions and units used in the study

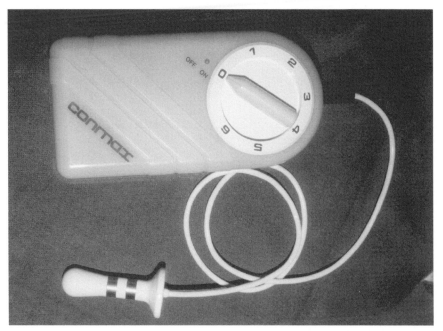

Figure 19.1. Electrical stimulator connected by a cable to the bipolar anal plug electrodes.

conformed with the International Continence Society (ICS) standards.[33] The Wilcoxon matched-pairs test was used for statistical evaluation.

Results

On average 12.4 months after the end of anal MES, sterile urine specimens were obtained from 23 (59%) of the 39 stimulated girls with recurrent UTI.

One month after the termination of anal MES the 23 cured girls demonstrated significantly changed cystometric parameters (Table 19.1). Typical inhibition of the detrusor, noted one month after the end of treatment with anal MES, is shown in Fig. 19.2.

In 13 girls in whom the therapy produced no improvement, no statistically significant changes in the studied cystometric parameters were found (Table 19.2).

Discussion

Various antibiotic agents used to treat UTI in children have proved quite ineffective. The failure of children with UTI to respond to antibiotic therapy may be due to unstable bladder, a condition found in 40–60% of these patients.[1,2] UTI may occur as a result of repeatedly elevated

Urodynamic variables	Before MES*	After MES*	p
First desire to void (ml)	85 (30–250)	120 (60–220)	NS[†]
Maximum cystometric capacity (ml)	240 (100–420)	300 (180–450)	≤0.001
Compliance	12 (2–70)	21 (2–80)	≤0.001
Number of unstable contractions	5 (1–22)	1 (1–13)	≤0.05

*Values are means (ranges in parentheses).
[†]NS, not significant.

Table 19.1. Urodynamic results before and after anal maximal electrical stimulation (MES) in 23 girls subsequently cured of recurrent urinary tract infection

intravesical pressure due to uninhibited contractions of the detrusor.[10,11,34] The management of the uninhibited bladder seems to reduce the risk of UTI.

In 1979, Koff et al.,[11] in their prospective uncontrolled study, gave anticholinergic medication to 52 children (48 girls and five boys) with unstable bladder and succeeded in sterilizing the urine in 58% of the patients.

In another study, Koff and Murtagh[12] treated, with antibiotics and oxybutinin, 62 neurologically normal children with UTI. Over a period of 6 years they achieved a sixfold decrease in the rate of UTI in this group compared with the controls, who had been treated with antibiotics alone.

Excellent results of treatment with anticholinergic drugs and antibiotics in patients with UTI were reported by Qvist et al:[35] 6 months after the termination of therapy, all the seven children treated were cured.

Hjalmas and Hellstrom,[36] who used a biofeedback method for the treatment of UTI and micturition problems in 56 children, reported 43 cures (77%) in 1–2 years.

Similar results have been obtained in the study reported here, with the application of ES in children with UTI and unstable bladder: the urine of 23 patients (59%) became sterile on average 12.4 months after the last MES application. Control urodynamic studies showed improvement of lower urinary tract function. A statistically significant increase was noted in the maximum cystometric capacity, compliance and volume of the first uninhibited contraction, together with a statistically significant decrease in the number of uninhibited contractions. These findings endorse the connection between UTI and unstable bladder.

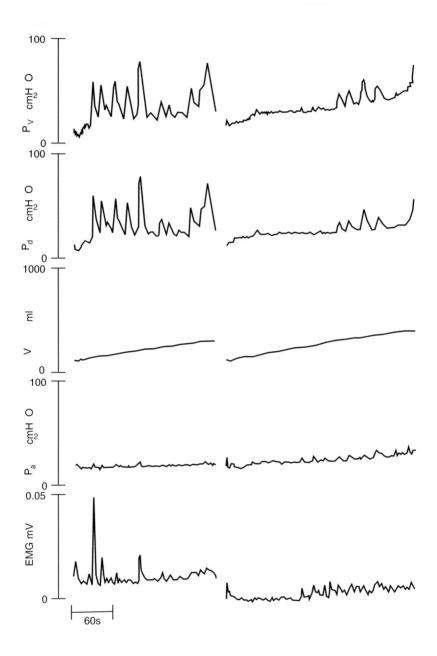

Figure 19.2. Cystometry before, and 4 months after, anal maximal electrical stimulation (MES) in an 11-year-old girl with recurrent lower urinary tract infection: EMG, electromyography of anal sphincter; P_a, abdominal pressure; P_d, detrusor pressure; P_v, vesical pressure; V, volume of bladder.

Urodynamic variables	Before MES*	After MES*	p
First desire to void (ml)	90 (50–160)	100 (60–140)	NS[†]
Maximum cystometric capacity (ml)	240 (150–370)	290 (200–350)	NS
Compliance	14 (5–33)	22 (6–59)	NS
Number of unstable contractions	3 (1–9)	2 (1–7)	NS

*,[†] As in Table 19.1.

Table 19.2. Urodynamic results before and after anal MES in 13 girls in whom recurrent urinary tract infection was not subsequently cured

In 13 girls, positive urine cultures persisted after the end of MES despite urinary antiseptic therapy. In this group, anal MES produced no significant change in the urodynamic parameters studied. This failure of ES may be explained by severe organic changes in the bladder wall, such as chronic cystitis and severe trabeculations.

Clearly, unstable bladder is only one of the possible causes of UTI in children who have no infravesical obstruction or neurogenic bladder. Other factors, such as the degree of virulence of bacteria, abnormal colonization of the periurethral aerobic flora in girls liable to UTI,[37] the degree of adhesiveness of Gram-negative urinary pathogens to human uroepithelial cells,[38] impaired local immune defence systems in the bladder wall[39] and the role of oestrogens in the binding of various bacteria to the epithelial cells,[40] have not been investigated in this study.

Conclusion

Anal MES can be recommended as an effective method for treating recurrent infections of the lower urinary tract and unstable bladder in children.

References

1. Bauer S B, Retik A B, Colodney A H et al. The unstable bladder of childhood. Urol Clin North Am 1980; 7: 321–336
2. Mayo M E, Burns M W. Urodynamic studies in children who wet. Br J Urol 1990; 65: 641–645
3. Palmatag H, Heering H, Ziegler G. Functional abnormality of 'non-provocative' bladder instability in children. Urol Int 1979; 34: 176–183
4. Nielsen J B, Djurhuus J C, Jorgensen T M. Lower urinary tract dysfunction in vesicoureteral reflux. Urol Int 1984; 39: 29–31

5. Artibani W, Ligato P, Bassi P *et al.* Detrusor overactivity in children and so-called primary vesicoureteral reflux. In: Proc 15th Meet Int Continence Soc, London, 1985; 294–295

6. Tršinar B. Urodinamske in klinične značilnosti idiopatskega otroškega nestabilnega mehurja. Zdrav Vestn 1992; 61: 17–21

7. Mehrotra R M L. An experimental study of the vesical circulation during distention and cystitis. J Pathol Bacteriol 1953; 66: 79

8. Finkbeiner A, Lapides J. Effects of distention on blood flow in dog's urinary bladder. Invest Urol 1974; 12: 210

9. Siroky B M, Nehra A, Vardi Y, Krane R J. Vesical blood flow: effect of hydrodistention and nerve stimulation. Neurourol Urodyn 1990; 9: 360–361

10. Parsons C L, Greenspan L, Moore C S W, Mulholland S G. Role of surface mucin in primary antibacterial defense of bladder. Urology 1977; 9: 48–52

11. Koff A S, Lapides J, Piazza H D. Association of urinary tract infection and reflux with uninhibited bladder contraction and voluntary sphincteric obstruction. J Urol 1979; 122: 373–376

12. Koff S A, Murtagh D S. The uninhibited bladder in children: effect of treatment on recurrence of urinary infection and on vesico-ureteral reflux resolution. J Urol 1983; 130: 1138–1141

13. Wein A J. Practical uropharmacology. Urol Clin North Am 1991; 18: 269–281

14. Thüroff J W, Bunke B, Ebner A *et al.* Randomized, double-blind multicenter trial on treatment of frequency, urgency and incontinence related to detrusor hyperactivity: oxybutinin vs. propantheline vs. placebo. Neurourol Urodynam 1990; 9: 336–337

15. Hellstrom A L, Hjalmas K, Jodal U. Terodiline in the treatment of children with unstable bladders. Br J Urol 1989; 63: 358–362

16. Jeffcoate T N, Francis W J. Urgency incontinence in the female. Am J Obstet Gynecol 1966; 94: 604–618

17. Cardozo L D, Abrams P D, Stanton S L. Idiopathic bladder instability treated by biofeedback. Br J Urol 1978; 50: 521–523

18. Millard R J, Oldenburg B. The symptomatic, urodynamic and psychodynamic results of bladder re-education programs. J Urol 1983; 130: 715–719

19. Cameron-Strange A, Millard R J. Management of refractory detrusor instability by transvesical phenol injection. Br J Urol 1988; 62: 323–325

20. Hamed H M, Sutherst J R, Richmond D H. The use of simple bladder distention in the treatment of detrusor instability. In: Proc 19th A Meet Int Continence Soc, Ljubljana, 1989: 194–195

21. Mundy A R. The long-term results of bladder transection for urge incontinence. Br J Urol 1983; 55: 642–644

22. Philp T, Shah P J R, Worth P H L. Acupuncture in the treatment of bladder instability. Br J Urol 1988; 61: 490–496

23. Pelvnik S, Janež J. Maximal electrical stimulation for urinary incontinence. Urology 1979; 14: 638–645

24. Fossberg E. Urge incontinence treated with maximal electric stimulation. Neurourol Urodyn 1988; 7: 270–271

25. Plevnik S. Electrical therapy. In: Stanton S L (ed) Clinical gynaecologic urology. St Louis: Mosby, 1984: 462–474

26. Sundin T, Carlsson C A. Reconstruction of several dorsal roots innervating the urinary bladder: an experimental study in cats. 1. Studies on the normal afferent pathways in the pelvic and pudendal nerves. Scand J Urol Nephrol 1972; 6: 176–184

27. Sundin T, Carlsson C A, Kock N G. Detrusor inhibition induced from mechanical

stimulation of the anal region and from electrical stimulation of pudendal nerve afferents. Invest Urol 1974; 11: 374–378

28. Lindstrom S, Fall M, Carlsson C A, Erlandson B E. The neurophysiological basis of bladder inhibition in response to intravaginal electrical stimulation. J Urol 1983; 129: 405–410

29. Vodušek D B, Light J K, Libby J M. Detrusor inhibition induced by stimulation of pudendal nerve afferents. Neurourol Urodyn 1986; 5: 381–389

30. Vodušek D B, Plevnik S, Vrtačnik P, Janež J. Detrusor inhibition on selective pudendal nerve stimulation in the perineum. Neurourol Urodyn 1988; 6: 389–393

31. Janež J. Električna stimulacija pri zdravljenju urinske inkontinence: mehanizmi delovanja. Doktorska disertacija, Medicinska fakulteta Univerze Edvarda Kardelja, Ljubljana, 1982

32. Janež J, Plevnik S, Korošec L et al. Changes in detrusor receptor activity after electric pelvic floor stimulation. In: Proc 11th A Meet Int Continence Soc, Lund, 1981: 22–23

33. International Continence Society. Fourth report on the standardisation of terminology of lower urinary tract function. Br J Urol; 51: 333–335

34. Kondo A, Kobayashi M, Otani T et al. Children with unstable bladder: clinical and urodynamic observation. J Urol 1983; 129: 88–91

35. Qvist N, Nielsen K K, Kristensen E S et al. Detrusor instability in children with recurrent urinary tract infection and/or enuresis. Urol Int 1986; 41: 199–201

36. Hjalmas K, Hellstrom A L. Habilitation of dysfunctional bladder in children. In: Proc 11th A Meet Int Continence Soc, Lund, 1981: 48–49

37. Bollgren I, Winberg J. The periurethral aerobic flora in girls highly susceptible to urinary tract infections. Acta Paediatr Scand 1976; 65: 81–87

38. Bruce A W, Chan R C Y, Pinkerton D et al. Adherence of Gram-negative urinary pathogens to human uroepithelial cells. J Urol 1983; 130: 293

39. Svanborg-Eden C, Svennerholm A M. Secretory immunoglobulin A and G antibodies prevent adhesion of Escherichia coli to human urinary tract epithelial cells. Infect Immun 1978; 22: 790–797

40. Botta G A. Possible role of hormones in the observed changes in adhesion of several microorganisms to epithelial cells from different body sites. FEMS Microbiol Lett 1981; 11: 69

Neurogenic voiding dysfunction in children with lumbosacral lipoma: can early neurosurgical intervention preserve voiding function?

20

T. Shibata S. Kobayashi H. Kakizaki
F. Takakura K. Ameda K. Matsumura
Y. Shinno T. Koyanagi

Introduction

Lumbosacral lipoma is the most common lesion in occult spinal dysraphism, which also includes conditions such as congenital dermal sinus, diastematomyelia and tight filum terminale, among others. It is usually concomitant with spinal cord tethering and causes insidious deterioration of sensorimotor nerve function and/or voiding and bowel function in children. It is believed that traction by the tethering, or compression by a lipoma, could lead to ischaemic damage and chronic inflammation in the spinal cord or nerve roots.[1] Many paediatric neurosurgeons have adopted a policy of early lipoma resection and release of the tethered cord for improvement of lower extremity malfunction or to prevent further impairment.[2-5] However, there is little information about the efficacy of neurosurgical intervention in preserving or regaining voiding function.[6-10] In order to evaluate the efficacy of early intervention for improvement of voiding function, therefore, the authors have retrospectively reviewed the clinical features and urodynamic data of 20 patients who underwent neurosurgical intervention for lumbosacral lipoma.

Patients and methods

The authors reviewed the urological evaluation and management of 20 patients (11 male and nine female) who underwent surgical resection of lumbosacral lipoma and release of tethered spinal cord between 1977 and 1993. Patients' ages at initial presentation ranged from 1 month to 16 years old (mean 4.2 years). The neurosurgical operation was performed when patients were between 1 month and 16 years old; nine patients underwent surgery when less than 1.5 years old; 11 were more than 1.5 years old at operation. All patients underwent urodynamic examination and spinal magnetic resonance imaging (MRI) or CT scan. Urodynamic testing was performed in all patients postoperatively and in ten preoperatively. External urethral sphincter electromyography (EUS-EMG) took place in 13 patients postoperatively, using a concentric needle electrode. In some patients this was performed under general anaesthesia, by a previously reported method.[11] Postoperative cystometry and voiding cystourethrography were performed on 19 and 20 patients, respectively. Postoperative urodynamic findings were compared between the groups in which neurosurgical intervention was undertaken before the age of 1.5 years or after 1.5 years of age. Diagnosis of neurogenic voiding dysfunction (NVD) was based on abnormal urodynamic findings, either presence of uninhibited contractions (UIC), with or without vesical denervation supersensitivity (Vds)[12] on cystometry, detrusor sphincter dyssynergia (DSD), and/or abnormal findings on voiding cystourethrography. Patients diagnosed as displaying NVD were placed on a programme of clean intermittent catheterization.

Results

Lumbosacral cutaneous lesions were confirmed to be present in 15 (94%) of 16 patients preoperatively: they comprised a subcutaneous mass in nine cases, skin dimple in seven, asymmetry of the hip in five, a patch of hair in two and a tail-like caudal appendage (human tail) in one. Sacral bone dysgenesis was found in 13 of 20 patients (65%), on plain radiography. A tethered cord was found in 17 patients (85%) on MRI or CT scan. Sensorimotor nerve abnormalities were found in six patients (30%); in five of these patients, surgical intervention took place after the age of 1.5 years.

Urodynamic findings are shown in Table 20.1. In the early surgical intervention group (before the age of 1.5 years), EUS-EMG and cystometry were normal in 83% (5/6) and 43% (3/7), respectively. A single case of DSD was later rediagnosed as non-NVD when normal voiding was confirmed. Voiding cystourethrography appeared to be

Group	Patient no.	Sex	Age (years:months)	CMG Pre	CMG Post	EMG Pre	EMG Post	VCU Pre	VCU Post	VF Pre	VF Post
Early	1	M	0:1	ND	Norm	ND	Norm	RU	RU	?	Norm
	2	F	0:4	ND	ND	ND	Norm	ND	VUR	?	Norm
	3	F	0:1	ND	UIC	ND	Norm	Norm	Norm	?	Norm
	4	M	0:6	ND	UIC	ND	ND	ND	RU, Deform	?	NVD
	5	M	0:2	ND	Norm	ND	Norm	ND	Norm	?	Norm
	6	M	0:7	ND	Norm	ND	Norm	ND	VUR	?	Norm
	7	M	1:3	ND	UIC Vds	ND	?	ND	VUR, Deform	?	NVD
	8	M	0:5	ND	UIC	ND	ND	ND	RU, VUR	?	NVD
	9	F	1:3	ND	Failed	ND	ND	ND	Norm	?	Norm
Late	1	M	10:0	UIC	Norm	Norm	Norm	Strain, VUR	Strain, VUR	NVD	NVD
	2	M	10:0	UIC	UIC	ND	DSD	ND	RU	?	NVD
	3	F	5:4	UIC, Vds	UIC	ND	ND	Deform, VUR, RU	Deform, VUR, RU	NVD	NVD
	4	M	4:0	?	Norm	ND	DSD	Deform, RU	Deform, RU	NVD	NVD
	5	F	9:0	UIC	UIC	DSD	ND	VUR	?	NVD	NVD
	6	M	9:0	UIC	UIC	DSD	DSD	No Void	No Void	NVD	NVD
	7	F	16:5	UIC, Vds	Norm	DSD	DSD	No Void	No Void	NVD	NVD
	8	F	1:10	ND	UIC, Vds	ND	ND	No Void, VUR	No Void, VUR	NVD	NVD
	9	M	1:9	ND	UIC	ND	ND	ND	Strain, RU	?	NVD
	10	F	2:5	ND	UIC	ND	DSD	ND	RU	?	NVD
	11	F	3:10	UIC	UIC	ND	DSD	No Void, VUR	No Void, VUR	NVD	NVD

*CMG, cystometrogram (ND, not done; Norm, normal; UIC, uninhibited contractions; Vds, vesical denervation supersensitivity); EMG, electromyography (DSD, detrusor sphincter dyssynergia); VCU, voiding cystourethrography (RU, residual urine; VUR, vesicoureteral reflux; Deform, bladder deformity; Strain, voiding on straining); VF, vesicourethral function (NVD, neurogenic voiding dysfunction).

Table 20.1. Urodynamic findings* before (Pre) and after (Post) surgical resection of lipoma and release of tethered spinal cord in 20 patients undergoing surgery before (early group) or after (late group) the age of 1.5 years

normal in 33% (3/9) and equivocal in 33% (3/9). Overall, three patients (33%) were diagnosed as NVD and placed on a programme of clean intermittent catheterization. On the other hand, in the late surgical intervention group (surgery after the age of 1.5 years), cystometry was normal in only three patients (27%) and EUS-EMG revealed DSD in 86% (6/7) postoperatively. In voiding cystourethrography, all patients had absent or poor urinary flow, with significant residual urine. All 11 patients in the late surgical intervention group were diagnosed as NVD and nine were placed on clean intermittent catheterization. There was a statistically significant difference in the incidence of postoperative NVD between the two groups ($p<0.01$, chi-square test).

Discussion

Lumbosacral lipoma is considered to be one of the components of occult spinal dysraphism and has been described as a rare but detectable cause of voiding dysfunction. After Bassett published a detailed study on lipomyelomeningocoele in 1950,[2] many paediatric neurosurgeons have advocated early surgical intervention for improvement or prevention of lower sensorimotor nerve malfunction.[3–5]

Few reports, however, have addressed specifically the efficacy of early neurosurgical intervention on the abolition or prophylaxis of urinary symptoms and/or urodynamic abnormality. Foster et al.[8] reported that, in 12 patients less than 1.5 years old at neurosurgical intervention, bladder function was normal preoperatively and postoperatively in five (42%) and normalized postoperatively in four (33%), whereas in 19 patients older than 1.5 years at operation, bladder function was normal both preoperatively and postoperatively in only four (21%), and became normal postoperatively in none.[8] They insisted that early neurosurgical intervention is mandatory for preservation of normal vesicourethral function, especially before the age of 1.5 years. According to Atala et al.,[9] in 29 patients undergoing surgery before the age of 15 months, preoperative urodynamic studies were abnormal in 11, and nine of 11 patients had excellent results postoperatively, whereas only one of six patients undergoing surgery between the ages of 4.5 and 19 years recovered normal vesicourethral function as determined by urodynamic studies.[9] Although the authors have insufficient preoperative urodynamic data, particularly in the early surgical intervention group, there is a statistically significant difference in the incidence of postoperative urodynamic abnormality between the early and late surgical intervention groups (33% vs 100%, $p<0.01$). In the early group it is not known whether postoperative normal vesicourethral function was brought about by the neurosurgical intervention or was already normal. Nevertheless, the rate of normal vesicourethral function in the early group was as high as 67% (6/9) postoperatively, which is consistent with the rate reported by Foster (75%).[8] The precise timing of the neurosurgical intervention has not yet been determined: previous reports advocated the operation after 1 year of age for reasons of technical feasibility and anaesthetic risk;[4] some recent reports, however, suggest that it should take place before the age of 6 months, because of the possibly high rate of recovery from sensorimotor malfunction.

Another factor that should be taken into account when considering early prophylactic operation is the possibility of neurological deficits developing postoperatively de novo as surgical complications. Atala *et al.* reported that one of 18 patients (6%) showed postoperative deterioration of urodynamic parameters.[9]

Chapman classified intraspinal lipomas into three types, according to their relationship to neural elements.[13] In 'transitional type' lipoma there is a complex relationship to the nerve roots and the spinal cord, so that it is difficult for neurosurgeons to resect them completely without damage to the neural elements; furthermore, lipoma itself causes a progressive deterioration in neural function. Hoffman stated that the fatty lump should not be regarded as a tumour and the aim of therapy should be the untethering of the spinal cord rather than the precise and accurate removal of all fat.[5] Great care must be taken to preclude surgical complications by leaving the neural elements undamaged.

In the authors' series, lumbosacral cutaneous lesions including subcutaneous mass, dimpling, hairy nevus, human tail or asymmetry, were detected in 94% of patients. Sacral bone dysgenesis was also detected radiographically in 65%. For early diagnosis in neonates and infants, a painstaking search for these subtle cutaneous lesions and for sacral bone dysgenesis, and an awareness of the association between underlying lumbosacral lipoma and congenital NVD, are essential before the advent of any urological deterioration. Careful and complete collaboration with obstetricians, paediatricians, orthopaedic surgeons, neurosurgeons and urologists is mandatory for the satisfactory management of these patients.

References

1. Yamada S, Zinke D E, Sanders D. Pathophysiology of 'tethered cord syndrome'. J Neurosurg 1981; 54: 494–503
2. Bassett R C. The neurological deficit associated with lipomas of the cauda equina. Ann Surg 1950; 131: 109–116
3. Swanson H S, Barnett J C. Intradural lipomas in children. Pediatrics 1962; 29: 911–926

4. Rogers H M, Long D M, Chou S N, French L A. Lipomas of the spinal cord and cauda equina. J Neurosurg 1971; 34: 349–354

5. Hoffman H J, Taecholarn C, Hendrick E B, Humphreys R P. Management of lipomyelomeningoceles. J Neurosurg 1985; 62: 1–8

6. Yoneyama T, Fukui J, Ohtsuka K et al. Urinary tract dysfunctions in tethered cord syndrome: improvement after surgical untethering. J Urol 1985; 133: 999–1001

7. Keating M A, Rink R C, Bauer S B et al. Neurourological implication of the changing approach in the management of occult spinal lesions. J Urol 1988; 140: 1299–1301

8. Foster L S, Kogan B A, Cogen P H, Edwards M S. Bladder function in patients with lipomyelomeningocele. J Urol 1990; 143: 984–986

9. Atala A, Bauer S B, Dyro F M et al. Bladder functional changes resulting from lipomyelomeningocele repair. J Urol 1992; 148: 592–594

10. Houle A M. Diastematomyelia and its neurourological implications. Dialogues in Pediatric Urology 1994; 17: 1–8

11. Ameda K, Kakizaki H, Kobayashi S et al. The evaluation of urodynamic study under general anesthesia for infants. Jpn J Urol 1993; 84: 975 (abstr)

12. Lapides J, Friend C R, Ajemian E P, Reus W F. A new test for neurogenic bladder. J Urol 1962; 88: 245–247

13. Chapman P H. Congenital intraspinal lipomas: anatomic considerations and surgical treatment. Childs Brain 1982; 9: 34–37

Rectus fascial sling for incontinence in male patients with myelodysplasia

21

A. K. Lee   K. M. Kim   D. K. Kim

Introduction

As children with myelodysplasia approach school age (4–5 years), there are increasing social and psychological pressures for them to be continent. Incontinence in patients with myelodysplasia may result from uninhibited bladder contractions, small bladder capacity, poor detrusor compliance, inadequate outlet resistance, or a combination of these factors. Approximately 95% of myelodysplastic children left untreated will be incontinent,[1] whereas a continence rate of 40–85% with a strict schedule of clean intermittent catheterization (CIC) and drugs (anticholinergics, imipramine, etc.) may be expected.[2–4] However, when all conservative measures are ineffective, an operation may be required.

The type of operation necessary to achieve continence depends on the size and cystometric characteristics of the bladder, the integrity of the urinary sphincter and the ability of the patient to perform self-catheterization. Ideally, all the procedures necessary to achieve continence should be performed in one operation. If the bladder is small or non-compliant, enlargement is necessary. Augmentation cystoplasty is a well-established method of improving storage capability. However, when the bladder neck is incompetent, a variety of options are available but none is uniformly applicable or successful.

One method whereby sphincter incompetence can be managed in girls with myelodysplasia is the fascial sling around the bladder neck and urethrae. Woodside and Borden[5] originally introduced its application in myelodysplasia and it has been performed successfully by many other urologists. In male patients, the periurethral sling procedure also can be carried out. McGuire, Raz, Elder and Decter have performed sling operations in male myelodysplastic patients and have reported their excellent results.[6–8]

The present authors have performed the fascial sling procedure in two male patients and the results are described in this chapter.

Case histories

Case 1

A 7 year-old boy presented with the chief complaint of urinary and faecal incontinence from birth. At birth he had a skin tag on his back, which was excised at the age of 1 year. No treatment other than simple excision was given. At the age of 6 years, owing to persistent urinary and faecal incontinence, he underwent spinal magnetic resonance imaging (MRI) and intravenous pyelography (IVP) in hospital. MRI showed a lumbosacral lipomeningomyelocoele with cord tethering and IVP showed mild upper tract dilatation with a trabeculated bladder. Suprapubic cystostomy was also conducted but urinary incontinence persisted. The patient was subsequently transferred to the authors' hospital. His urinalysis was clear and serum creatinine was within the normal range. Further urological work-ups included voiding cystourethrography (VCU) and urodynamic studies. A bladder neck widely opened in the resting state and no vesicoureteral reflux was found on VCU (Fig. 21.1). Cystometry via the suprapubic cystostomy tract revealed a hypertonic

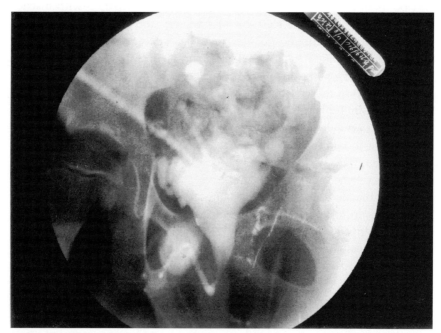

Figure 21.1. Preoperative cystogram demonstrating bladder neck wide open in the resting state (case 1).

bladder with poor compliance; urine leaking was observed after a 50 ml fluid infusion. Persistence of the gaping bladder neck was found on fluoroscopic monitoring, indicating an incompetent internal urethra sphincter. L5 laminoplastic laminectomy, debulking of intraspinal lipoma and untethering of the thickened filum terminale took place in the neurosurgical department. The patient was readmitted for reconstructive surgery of the lower urinary tract. Augmentation ileocystoplasy and the rectus fascial sling operation were performed. The bladder was augmented using a detubularized ileal segment (30 cm). The sling operation incorporated a modification of the McGuire/Raz approach.[6] The distal prostatic urethra was suspended using a rectus fascial segment (1.5 × 10 cm), each end of which was sutured to the ipsilateral Cooper's ligament with no. 1 prolene. The postoperative period was unremarkable. Catheter drainage was maintained for 3 weeks and cystography after catheter removal revealed increased bladder capacity with a closed proximal urethra (Fig. 21.2). A follow-up urodynamic study 3 months postoperatively showed a bladder with good compliance up to 200 ml filling volume. During the course of a 1-year follow-up, the patient has been completely dry with CIC five times daily.

Case 2

An 11 year-old boy presented with the chief complaint of urinary and faecal incontinence, which had also led to troublesome recurrent perineal eczema. At birth his parents noted a low back mass and foot

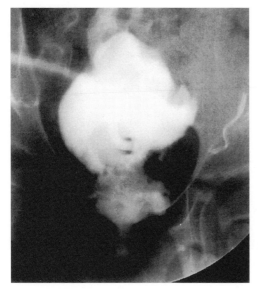

Figure 21.2. Postoperative cystogram demonstrating increased bladder capacity with closed proximal urethra (case 1).

deformity: the diagnosis was lumbosacral meningomyelocoele with hydrocephalus and bilateral equinovarus. At the age of 7 months he received a ventriculoperitoneal shunt and meningomyelocoele repair operation. At the age of 11, a triple arthrodesis for the correction of the foot deformity was carried out in the authors' hospital. Following his presentation to the Department of Urology for the urinary incontinence persisting from birth, a urological work-up included urinalysis, urine culture, serum chemistry, IVP, VCU and urodynamic study. Urinalysis showed the presence of pyuria and the urine culture was positive for *Escherichia coli*. The serum creatinine level was within the normal range. IVP and VCU showed a moderate degree of upper tract dilatation (right<left) with bilateral grade II/III VUR (Fig. 21.3). On cystometry, there were uninhibited contractions during bladder filling and the functional bladder capacity was less than 100 ml. A persistently opened bladder neck was found in fluoroscopic monitoring during cystometry, regardless of uninhibited contraction. It was decided to construct an umbilical stoma for self-catheterization because the patient was on crutches owing to his orthopaedic problems. Reconstructive surgery of the lower urinary tract was therefore planned, as follows: augmentation gastrocystoplasty; bilateral ureteral reimplantation; stoma formation using the appendix (Mitrofanoff procedure), rectus fascial sling operation

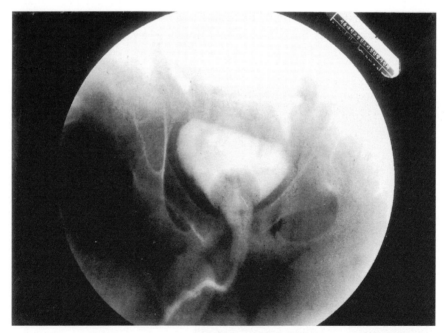

Figure 21.3. Preoperative cystogram demonstrating bladder neck wide open in the resting state, and bilateral vesicoureteral reflux (case 2).

(modified McGuire/Raz approach). A triangular segment (9 × 9 × 12 cm) was mobilized in the body of the stomach for augmentation gastrocystoplasty. Each ureter was reimplanted on the lateral side of an ipsilateral wedge flap of stomach segment with a submucosal tunnel 3 cm long. A pedicled flap including the distal portion of the caecum and appendix was mobilized. The appendiceal portion was reimplanted on the dome side of the stomach segment with a submucosal tunnel 2 cm long and the caecum portion of the flap was anastomosed with the umbilicus to form the stoma. A rectus fascial sling operation was performed as described for case 1. Three weeks postoperatively, the catheter was removed and intermittent catheterization was started via the appendicovesicostomy tract. Postoperative IVP and VCU showed decreased upper urinary tract dilatation and increased bladder capacity with no VUR, but coaptation of the proximal urethra was incomplete (Fig. 21.4). A urodynamic study 3 months postoperatively showed good bladder compliance with over 250 ml of functional bladder capacity and no uninhibited contractions. During 10 months follow-up with CIC via the appendicovesicostomy tract, intermittent wetting through the urethra persisted, but in small amounts. The patient is now free from his longstanding perineal eczema.

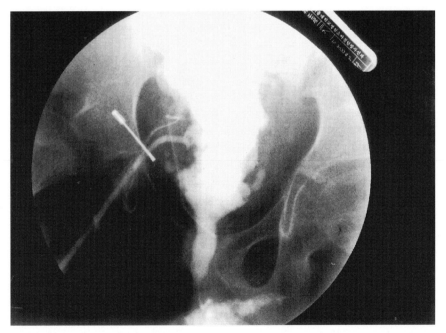

Figure 21.4. Postoperative cystogram demonstrating increased bladder capacity with no vesicoureteral reflux, but incomplete coaptation of the proximal urethra (case 2).

Discussion

The most common operation in male patients with refractory sphincter incompetence from myelodysplasia is the construction of an artificial sphincter.[9,10] Although urinary incontinence is completely prevented, approximately 50% of those with an artificial sphincter and an augmented bladder have to perform CIC to drain the bladder completely.[11]

Long-term follow-up studies by Bosco and associates have demonstrated that 69% of sphincters implanted (25 of 36) were still functioning properly after 5 years. However, 40% of functioning sphincters (10 of 25) had required one further operation, because of mechanical complications and ischaemic atrophy of the urethra.[9] A recent report showed shedding of silicone particles from the device in two of five patients who had the sphincter in place for a mean of 5.5 years. Whether there is any long-term hazard associated with these particles is unknown.[12]

A popular method in myelodysplastic girls has been the periurethral or pubovaginal sling, in which a free graft of rectus fasica is placed around the bladder neck, suspending it to the rectus fascia or pubic symphysis.[13,14]

In male patients, a periurethral sling can also be carried out. Raz and associates reported four cases in which this surgical approach was used in male patients with meningomyelocoele who were suffering from severe urinary incontinence attributable to poor bladder compliance and sphincter incompetence.[6] Raz and associates took the sling from the rectus sheath, leaving the base of the strip attached to the fascia while the other end was placed around the urethra as a free graft. The sling was located beneath the distal prostatic urethra and the tension on the sling was determined somewhat empirically. Those authors consider that the goal is to obtain coaptation and compression of the incompetent and paralysed proximal urethra. The increase in pressure in the proximal urethra was about 6–12 cmH$_2$O, but with coughing and straining the closing pressure increased markedly because of the action of the sling.

In the present authors' opinion, assessment of the outlet in myelodysplastic patients is the most difficult aspect of the evaluation. They perform the sling procedure concomitantly with augmentation cystoplasty in cases where a wide open bladder neck and low intravesical pressures at the time of leakage are revealed by videourodynamic studies. The technique is similar to that of Raz because it is not easy to place the sling around the bladder neck in male patients. One patient was totally dry at 1-year follow-up, but the other patient had complained of stress incontinence for 10 months of follow-up. In the latter this wetting was probably due to a technical error of sling placement: the sling was positioned too distal to the bladder neck and less tightly attached. Elder and Decter position the sling around the bladder neck and increase the tension on the sling until no leakage occurs on vigorous manipulation of the full bladder by the operator.[7,8] However, in the Decter's series, catheterization difficulty developed in three patients. In that author's opinion, this is due to varying degrees of erosion of the sling, and it is better to adjust the fascial tension so that it stops leakage of the fully distended bladder on gentle manipulation.[8] Modifying the technique of adjusting the sling tension and positioning the sling is one of the problems awaiting solution associated with the sling operation in male patients.

In conclusion, the periurethral sling operation appears to be an excellent alternative to the artificial sphincter in properly selected male patients with myelodysplasia, but further experience and longer follow-up are needed for a complete assessment of this procedure.

References

1. Lorber J, Salfield S A. Results of selective treatment of spina bifida cystica. Arch Dis Child 1981; 56: 822–830
2. Cass A S, Luxenberg M, Johnson C F. Management of the neurogenic bladder in 413 children. J Urol 1984; 132: 521–525
3. Kaplan W E. Management of the urinary tract in myelomeningocele. Probl Urol 1988; 2: 121
4. Purcell M H, Gregory J G. Intermittent catheterization: evaluation of complete dryness and independence in children with myelomeningocele. J Urol 1984; 132: 518–520
5. Woodside J R, Borden T A. Pubovaginal sling procedure for the management of urinary continence in a myelodysplastic girl. J Urol 1982; 127: 744–746
6. Raz S, McGuire E J, Ehrlich RM et al. Fascial sling to correct male neurogenic sphincter incompetence: the McGuire/Raz approach. J Urol 1988; 139: 528–531
7. Elder J S. Periurethral and puboprostatic sling repair for incontinence in patients with myelodysplasia. J Urol 1990; 144: 434–437
8. Decter R M. Use of the fascial sling for neurogenic incontinence: lessons learned. J Urol 1993; 150: 683–686
9. Bosco P J, Bauer S B, Colodny A H. The longterm results of artificial sphincters in children. J Urol 1991; 146: 396–399
10. Sidi A A, Reinberg Y, Gonzalez R. Comparison of artificial sphincter implantation and bladder neck reconstruction in patients with neurogenic urinary incontinence. J Urol 1987; 138: 1120–1122
11. Rink R C, Mitchell M E. Bladder neck/urethral reconstruction in the neuropathic bladder. Dialogues Pediatr Urol 1987; 10: 5
12. Reinberg Y, Manivel J C, Gonzalez R. Silicone shedding from artificial urinary sphincter in children. Presented at the Annual Meeting, Urology Section, American Academy of Pediatrics 1992; October

13. Bauer S B, Peters C A, Colodny A H. The use of rectus fascia to manage urinary incontinence. J Urol 1989; 142: 516–519
14. McGuire E J, Wang C C, Usitalo H, Savastano J. Modified pubovaginal sling in girls with myelodysplasia. J Urol 1986; 135: 94–96

Enterocystoplasty without bladder neck surgery for the myelodysplastic patient requiring bladder augmentation

22

T. D. Allen   M. L. Cher   D. H. Ewalt

Introduction

Historically, urological interest in the myelodysplastic patient has centred primarily around the urinary incontinence attributed to intrinsic urethral sphincter deficiency, and to treat this incontinence, a variety of procedures have been offered to increase outlet resistance.[1–4] More recent investigations into the pathophysiology of this problem, however, have suggested that wetness in these patients is not so much a matter of failure to hold as failure to store, and currently the emphasis has shifted to establishing a large-volume low-pressure bladder reservoir. Nevertheless, the swing to bladder augmentation procedures to accomplish this goal has not been accompanied by an equivalent loss of enthusiasm for procedures on the bladder neck. Many investigators still believe that, even with vesical augmentation, there is a continued need for increasing outlet resistance if dryness is to be assured.[5,6]

The authors' feelings have been somewhat different. In a review of their own experience with vesical augmentation for the incontinent myelodysplastic patient, they concluded that, if ileocystoplasty is done, no procedure is necessary for the bladder neck, provided that outlet resistance is at least 30 cmH$_2$O. This current report, extending the series to 30 patients, confirms the rationale of such a philosophy.

Patients and methods

Since mid-1986 the authors have performed ileocystoplasty on 30 myelodysplastic patients with reservoir inadequacy in the absence of a history of previous surgery on the bladder neck or urethra. Sixteen of these patients have been reported previously.[7] The series encompasses 23 patients with myelomeningocoele, four with sacral malformation and three with sacral lipoma associated with tethered cord; there were ten male and 20 female patients. Their ages ranged from 2 to 18 years, except for one man who was 28 years old. Fifteen were ambulatory, four walked with braces or crutches, and 11 were wheelchair bound. All had inadequate bladder storage capacity as suggested by wetness despite clean intermittent catheterization (CIC), increasing hydronephrosis, vesicoureteral reflux, rising creatinine, or recurrent urinary tract infection. Twenty-two were on CIC prior to the augmentation: four went from vesicostomy and one from ureterostomy directly to augmentation, and three others went directly from an intact bladder to augmentation without a preliminary trial of CIC. The patients were consecutive and all inclusive with one exception, a girl with no measurable outlet resistance at all who went elsewhere for placement of an artificial sphincter.

All patients underwent urodynamic studies preoperatively which included a cystometrogram, a leak-point pressure (LPP) or urethral pressure profile (UPP) and, more recently, electromyography. Inadequate bladder storage capacity was confirmed by the findings of a safe volume (volume at pressures below 30 cmH$_2$O) inadequate to permit a 4-hourly catheterization schedule at expected levels of urinary output. UPP and LPP were determined using an 8 Fr catheter initially and a 7 Fr catheter more recently. Although there was some variation in the results encountered with different techniques, the values in the same patient were similar. Overall outlet resistance in these patients ranged from 19 to more than 100 cmH$_2$O, averaging 54 cmH$_2$O (Fig. 22.1). In only one patient, however, was urethral resistance consistently below 30 cmH$_2$O.

All patients underwent ileocystoplasty by the technique described by Goodwin et al.,[8] using approximately 40 cm of distal ileum. A Mitrofanoff-type entry into the bladder using the appendix was constructed at the same time in three patients to allow for easier catheterization, and eight patients also underwent ureteral reimplantation at the time of the augmentation. Nothing was done to the bladder neck or urethra to increase outlet resistance in any patient, regardless of the urodynamic findings.

Results

There were no deaths in the series, and preoperative hydronephrosis and elevated creatinine improved or stabilized in all patients. One patient subsequently underwent operation for intestinal obstruction, one suffered a wound dehiscence requiring secondary closure, and in one a Mitrofanoff-type entry to the bladder was subsequently constructed, using a segment of ureter when his urethra strictured, possibly because of

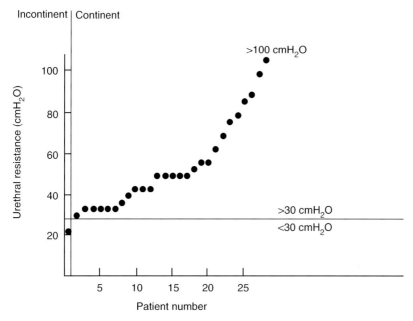

Figure 22.1. Graph of individual urethral resistances laid out in ascending order. The values for two patients are no longer available. The only patient with incontinence after ileocystoplasty was the one patient with a urethral resistance of less than 30 cmH₂O.

an allergy to latex. One patient had an episode subsequently that may have represented a spontaneous rupture of the augment, but this happened elsewhere and the aetiology of the event was never confirmed. Two patients later formed bladder stones requiring removal. Problems with urinary tract infection following the augmentation were usually minor and generally secondary to flaws in the technical aspect of the catheterization (too small a catheter, failure to adhere to a proper catheterization schedule, failure to empty the bladder completely, failure to flush out mucus periodically, etc). Minor degrees of hyperchloraemic acidosis were seen in patients with marginal renal function but were easy to control.

All the patients are now completely dry on 4-hourly CIC during the day, regardless of activity, except the one with an outlet resistance of only 19–22 cmH₂O. He exhibited stress incontinence and was consequently offered an artificial sphincter, but the family declined the surgery. He was seen several years later with an outlet resistance that had risen to 30 cmH₂O and was completely dry except when he strained while playing the trumpet. Several patients noted dampness or wetness during sleep if they did not catheterize themselves once during the night, but most made it through the night without catheterization and remained dry.

Discussion

As is evident from this expanded series, the authors' experience continues to show that an outlet resistance equal to or exceeding 30 cmH$_2$O is adequate in itself to ensure dryness in the myelodysplastic patient on a 4-hourly catheterization schedule following ileocystoplasty. Admittedly, it could be argued that the series might be biased by the fact that most of these patients exhibited impaired bladder compliance, suggesting straining against a resistance, and that, therefore, it might not be an accurate reflection of the full spectrum of myelodysplastic patients, many of whom might have a very low outlet resistance. Investigation, however, has failed to discover many patients with an outlet resistance below 30 cmH$_2$O, despite the authors' conscientious study of all patients with urinary incontinence. At the moment, it is their impression that myelodysplastic patients with an outlet resistance below 30 cmH$_2$O constitute less than 5% of the overall pool of these patients. Clearly, the need for bladder neck surgery in the myelodysplastic patient undergoing enterocystoplasty has been seriously overstated.

It is also noteworthy that the continence achieved in these patients is generally resistant to the effects of straining. This should not be so surprising, perhaps, in view of the recent investigations by McGuire et al.,[9] regarding the impact of intra-abdominal pressure upon the urinary tract in different clinical settings. Urinary incontinence, after all, represents nothing more than an excess of bladder pressure over urethral resistance. Unlike the urethra of the female with stress incontinence secondary to decensus of the bladder base, the bladder neck and proximal urethra of the myelodysplastic patient remain within the sphere of influence of the intra-abdominal pressure, and the pressure rise produced by straining affects both bladder and urethra equally. As the pressure within the bivalved bladder augmented with detubularized ileum seldom exceeds 20 cmH$_2$O at normal volumes, a urethral resistance of 30 cmH$_2$O is sufficient to prevent urinary leakage during all normal activity.

The same results may not be duplicated by colocystoplasty or gastrocystoplasty, even though colon and stomach appear to be the more popular structures used for augmentation in some series.[5,10,11] The amount of material available from the colon or stomach for use in augmentation is somewhat less and the walls of both are thicker, so that low-pressure distension is not as readily achieved as with ileum. In the authors' earlier experience using colon, dampness was noted in several such patients, and Rink *et al.*,[12] in reporting on persistent wetness in eight of 250 patients undergoing a variety of enterocystoplasties, noted that six of these were cases of colocystoplasty and two were cases of gastrocystoplasty; no cases of ileocystoplasty were involved.

Avoidance of surgery upon the bladder outlet may yield some additional benefits in these patients. As no reconstruction of the bladder neck has taken place, these patients are easy to catheterize, and the absence of an artificial sphincter has enabled concern for the mechanical breakdown and erosion problems that are associated with these devices to be avoided. Finally, an unoperated bladder outlet may serve as a safety valve allowing overflow through the urethra before rupture of the augment. The low incidence of spontaneous augment rupture noted in this series tends to support this belief.

Conversely, the demonstrated ability of bladder outlets of even marginal quality to provide continence in the myelodysplastic patient after ileocystoplasty emphasizes the importance of preserving this mechanism. Procedures designed to reduce this resistance in infancy and childhood in order to lessen the likelihood of developing poor bladder compliance[13] may exact a heavy price in later years if continence can no longer be achieved by simple ileocystoplasty.

In summary, the authors' experience with vesical augmentation using ileum alone in patients with congenital spinal disorders has now grown to 30 consecutive cases. Despite the fact that nothing was done to increase outlet resistance, all patients with a preoperative urethral resistance of 30 cmH$_2$O or more (all but one patient in the series) are now dry during the day on CIC. Avoidance of procedures upon the bladder neck has reduced late complications to a minimum, and has obviated the problem of spontaneous rupture of the augment. This precious urethral resistance, deficient as it may be in these patients, should be preserved in early life in case it is needed at a later stage.

References

1. Scott F B, Bradley W E, Timm G W, Kothari D. Treatment of incontinence secondary to myelodysplasia by an implantable prosthetic urinary sphincter. South Med J 1973; 66: 987–990
2. Leadbetter G W. Surgical correction of total urinary incontinence. J Urol 1964; 91: 261–266
3. Kropp K A, Angwafo F F. Urethral lengthening and reimplantation for neurogenic incontinence in children. J Urol 1986; 135: 533–536
4. McGuire E J, Wang C C, Usitalo H, Savastano J. Modified pubovaginal sling in girls with myelodysplasia. J Urol 1986; 135: 94–96
5. Bauer S B, Hendren W H, Kozakewich H et al. Perforation of the augmented bladder. J Urol 1992; 148: 699–703

6. Gonzalez R, Koleilat N, Austin C, Sidi A A. The artificial sphincter AS800 in congenital urinary incontinence. J Urol 1989; 142: 512–515

7. Cher M L, Allen T D. Continence in the myelodysplastic patient following enterocystoplasty. J Urol 1993; 149: 1103–1106

8. Goodwin W, Winter C C, Barker W F. 'Cup-patch' technique of ileocystoplasty for bladder enlargement or partial substitution. Surg Gynecol Obstet 1959; 108: 240

9. McGuire E J, Fitzpatrick C C, Wan J et al. Clinical assessment of urethral sphincter function. J Urol 1993; 150: 1452–1454

10. Mitchell M E, Kulb T B, Backes D J. Intestinocystoplasty in combination with clean intermittent catheterization in the management of vesical dysfunction. J Urol 1986; 136: 288–291

11. Kreder K J, Webster G D. Management of the bladder outlet in patients requiring enterocystoplasty. J Urol 1992; 147: 38–41

12. Rink R C, Keating M A, Adams M C. Augmenting the augmented bladder: addressing persistent incontinence. Presented to the American Academy of Pediatrics, Urology Section, New Orleans, Louisiana, 27 October 1991

13. Bloom D A, Knechtel J M, McGuire E J. Urethral dilation improves bladder compliance in children with myelomeningocele and high leak point pressures. J Urol 1990; 144: 430–433

Surgical treatment of urinary incontinence in children and adolescents with neuropathic bladder

23

J. Dvořáček   R. Kočvara   Z. Dítě
L. Jarolím

Introduction

Neurogenic or neuropathic bladder in the widest sense is an abnormality characterized by vesicourethral dysfunction resulting from a variety of diseases. The conditions producing neuropathic bladder may be congenital or acquired and of urological or non-urological nature. Some are obvious (such as myelomeningocoele), whereas others are occult and discovered only after thoughtful consideration and thorough investigation. The alteration in the micturition cycle, presented by urinary incontinence, and the risk of upper urinary tract deterioration, differ from case to case and depend on the underlying disease. Meningomyelocoele is one of the most common anomalies responsible for neuropathic bladder in children and adolescents.[1] Bladder exstrophy and posterior urethral valves in boys have a similar presentation and therapeutic strategy. Medical treatment, including clean intermittent catheterization (CIC) and anticholinergic therapy, fails in many patients suffering from neuropathic bladder.[2] These individuals, with non-compliant, high-pressure and small-capacity bladders, require bladder augmentation accompanied by other procedures to restore urinary continence.

The aim of surgery is to obtain a continent reservoir, with a large capacity low pressure and adequate urethral resistance. The achievement of this goal is a unique challenge that often necessitates subsequent complex surgical procedures. Unfortunately, some patients need both surgical and non-surgical therapy. A range of procedures for continent urinary reconstruction have been proposed; however, not all of these methods are suitable for young individuals.[3] Enterocystoplasty and gastrocystoplasty are currently well-established means of dealing with a non-compliant small-capacity high-pressure urinary bladder.[4-6] On the other hand, in spite of numerous reported options for continent reconstruction, the optimal method of urethral closure remains questionable, especially in the young. Bladder neck reconstruction according to Young–Dees–Leadbetter,[6] or a procedure creating a valve mechanism at the bladder neck,[7] should be the initial treatment. Some authors consider placement of an artificial sphincter as an alternative.[8,9] In some boys and disabled patients, CIC can be difficult or painful. Continent appendicovesicostomy[10] and its modifications[11–13] offer a solution to this situation. In view of these facts, an individual approach should be selected in most cases. The choice of therapeutic strategy is extremely important in children and adolescents with regard to their growth and life expectancy. In this chapter the authors' initial results are presented and their experience with the current trends in this field are discussed.

Patients and methods

From January 1991 to June 1994, 26 patients (16 male and ten female, ranging in age from 5 to 22 years, with a mean age of 14.2 years) underwent surgical intervention for neuropathic bladder at the authors' clinic. Patients underwent routine neurological and urological evaluation. Urodynamic evaluation [pressure–flow study, residual urine quantification, electromyography (facultatively on suspicion of dyssynergia) and urethral pressure profilometry] revealed urodynamic characteristics of involuntary bladder contractions (detrusor instability or hyperreflexia) in all patients, detrusor–sphincter dyssynergia in 12, and an incompetent or absent sphincter in 25 patients. The actual bladder volume and end filling pressure at capacity were recorded; the values were obtained by determining the capacity by cystometry at either the first desire to void or the point at which pain or urine leakage occurred.

The neuropathic bladder resulted from myelomeningocoele in 20 patients (77%), exstrophy–epispadias complex in two and posterior urethral valves in two boys. Voiding dysfunction and poorly detectable neurological abnormality were found in two patients, probably representing variants of the Hinman syndrome ('non-neurogenic neurogenic bladder').[14] The majority of patients experienced recurrent urinary tract infection (UTI) and 22 (85%) had positive urine cultures. Nineteen patients had vesicoureteral reflux (37/52 ureters or 71%) and dilatation of the upper urinary tract was established in 18 patients (69%). All patients were incontinent and attempts at medical management based on urodynamic findings had failed.

Detubularized augmentation ('clam')[15] ileocystoplasty was performed in 21 patients, colocystoplasty in three and gastrocystoplasty in the remaining two. Continence procedures performed in conjunction with augmentation cystoplasties included Mitrofanoff's continent appendicovesicostomy in ten children (in one boy the distal end of the right ureter was converted into a catheterizable stoma), Young–Dees– Leadbetter or Turner–Warwick bladder neck tubularization (the latter technique was preferred in the last final seven of 12 children), the Kropp urethral lengthening-reimplantation operation in one girl, and bladder neck suspension in four. The choice of procedure to increase urethral resistance was dictated by the function of the bladder neck and urethra of the individual patient. An artificial sphincter (AMS 800) was implanted in one boy and in two male adolescents. The device was placed twice around the bladder neck and once around the bulbous urethra. The AMS 800 was reserved for those older patients who were able to operate the sphincter dependably and who could empty the bladder completely.

Vesicoureteral reflux was corrected with a Cohen technique simultaneously in 16/37 (43%) ureteral units. Hospital stay ranged from 17 to 34 days (mean 22 days).

Results

There were no deaths. All patients were seen for follow-up after 1 and 6 months and then at regular intervals, dictated by the clinical course. The follow-up period ranged from 2 to 42 months (mean 24.3 months).

One early and two late complications (11%) were noted. A 12-year-old girl with an obstructive ileus required an adhesiectomy on postoperative day 9. A 17-year-old boy was readmitted 2 months after the uncomplicated surgery and postoperative course, with voiding difficulties caused by mucosal necrosis of the 'clam' segment. A year later he underwent a reintervention and gastrocystoplasty with Mitrofanoff stoma for persistent incontinence and a small non-compliant bladder. The third patient, a 15-year-old girl, presented with acute pyelonephritis and upper urinary tract dilatation secondary to ureterovesical stricture on the right side 2 years after the ileal clam augmentation and Kropp bladder neck procedure. The underlying aetiology was a non-compliant bladder with total urinary incontinence resulting from primary reconstruction of bladder exstrophy and bilateral antireflux Cohen procedures undergone at another institution as a neonate. The authors initially inserted a nephrostomy tube and, 4 weeks later, carried out a ureteral neoimplantation into the ileal clam using Le Duc's open-end technique.

Renal function remained improved or stable in all but one girl with impaired renal function occurring just prior to surgery. Analysis of urine culture revealed a significant decrease in the incidence of UTI (from 85 to 30%). In four patients significant cystitis or pyelonephritis required readmission. Eleven children take supplementary bicarbonate to correct metabolic acidosis. Comparison of the preoperative and postoperative cystograms demonstrated a significant increase in the mean relative volume (202%) in all cases. The actual bladder volume increased, from 70–250 ml (mean 125 ml) preoperatively to 195–720 ml (mean 377 ml) after intervention. The end filling pressure prior to reconstruction ranged from 31 to 68 cmH$_2$O (mean 52 cmH$_2$O) with uninhibited contractions in most cases. Postoperative follow-up examination revealed a fall in these parameters to an average of 22.3 cmH$_2$O (range 11–52 cmH$_2$O). In 12 patients persistent bladder instability was recorded in spite of successful surgery; this resolved on administration of anticholinergic drugs. The upper urinary tract dilatation confirmed preoperatively in 18 cases was abolished or improved in 12 patients (67%), remained unchanged in five (28%) and progressed in the remaining patient. Twenty-two patients practise CIC every 4–6 hours, and four (without reflux) urinate using Valsalva's and Crede's voiding techniques in combination. Of the 26 patients undergoing surgery for neuropathic bladder, 19 (73%) are continent by day and night using only one continence pad, if any; they are able to carry out physical activities such as coughing, laughing, and carrying or lifting weights, without loss of urinary continence; six (23%) have to use up to three pads a day and occasionally observe leakage at night and the final patient remains incontinent.

Discussion

Neuropathic bladder remains a topical subject despite recent advances in diagnosis as well as new possibilities in medical and surgical treatment, especially for the younger generation. Medical efforts are concentrated on two problems — to achieve urinary continence and to save the patient from upper urinary tract deterioration. Urinary incontinence in children and young adults is a severe social and physical burden. A variety of conservative and surgical means are currently available.

Urinary diversion, which has been so popular in recent times, is now regarded as outdated. Long-term follow-up in patients who have undergone supravesical diversion has been disappointing because of the significant incidence of renal deterioration, pyelonephritis and stone disease, and this procedure has been abandoned.[16] Since CIC was popularized by Lapides[2] (eliminating problems caused by inefficient voiding), it has come to be used in conjunction with new drugs (anticholinergics, alpha-sympathomimetics and antispasmodics) as a useful means of managing patients with neuropathic bladder. If these relatively simple means fail to achieve continence, surgery in combination with medical therapy is required. Today, a whole range of surgical techniques are used for the reconstruction of neuropathic bladder, including bladder enlargement, the Mainz pouch II[17] and continence restoring procedures; unfortunately, none of these is universally applicable and effective. Clam ileal augmentation appears to be the most popular method by which to achieve a large compliant urinary reservoir. Using the bowel to augment the bladder has recognized complications that occasionally may be quite severe, including electrolyte disturbance, production of mucus, enteric fistula abscess, peritoneal adhesions and urinary incontinence due to contractions of the bowel segment. These disadvantages are largely solved by gastrocystoplasty. The most recent trend is to use the DAWG technique (demucosalized auto-augmentation with gastric tissue), meaning the use of a denuded stomach muscle with bladder auto-augmentation, creating a full-thickness urothelial graft to the raw inner surface of incorporated stomach muscle.[18] The choice of the various alternative reconstruction procedures for the restoration of urinary continence continues to be open; most authors prefer procedures that increase outlet resistance (mostly the Young–Dees–Leadbetter, Turner-Warwick and Kropp techniques) over the artificial sphincters. Unfortunately, there are certain limitations to the use of CIC: some patients are unable to catheterize themselves because of orthopaedic problems, spasticity, wheelchair existence, leg braces, obesity or limited intellect. Some male patients find CIC on a frequent basis too irritating for acceptance. The Mitrofanoff continent appendicovesicostomy remains an option for these individuals.[11–13,19]

Despite this progress, the management of neuropathic bladder continues to be speculative. This is also confirmed by the great deal of attention devoted to this topic in the literature and at congress. The therapeutic strategy of neuropathic bladder should start with accurate diagnosis, mainly based on urodynamic evaluation. The patient's ability to perform CIC should be demonstrated before any augmentation cystoplasty. The choice of surgical strategy should be based on the patient's age and anatomical situation, as well as the personal experience of the surgeon. The importance of the general state of health and mentality of the patient should never be underestimated.

In this series the authors achieved urinary continence in 73% of their patients, renal function remained stable or improved in 96% and in 67% of cases the upper urinary tract dilatation was abolished or improved. These results are consistent with rates reported previously.[4,7,8,12,16,17]

From these findings it can be concluded that, in the majority of cases, concentrated attention devoted to patients with this condition brings about substantial improvement in their quality of life.

References

1. Bauer S B. Neurogenic bladder dysfunction. Pediatr Clin North Am 1987; 34: 1121–1132
2. Lapides J, Diokno A C, Silber S J, Lowe B S. Clean intermittent self-catheterization in the treatment of urinary tract disease. J Urol 1972; 107: 458–461
3. Gleeson M J, Griffith D P. Urinary diversion — review. Br J Urol 1990; 66: 113–122
4. Mitchell M E, Piser J A. Intestinocystoplasty and total bladder replacement in children and young adults: followup in 129 cases. J Urol 1987; 138: 579–584
5. Mundy A R. Neuropathic vesicourethral dysfunction. In: Mundy A R (ed) Urodynamic and reconstructive surgery of the lower urinary tract. London: Churchill Livingstone, 1993; 153–182
6. Simfest J M, Mitchell M E. Gastrocystoplasty in children. Eur Urol 1992; 5: 89–93
7. Kropp A K, Angwafo F F. Urethral lengthening and reimplantation for neurogenic incontinence in children. J Urol 1986; 135: 533–536
8. Gonzales R, Koleilat N, Austin C, Sidi A A. The artificial sphincter AS 800 in congenital urinary incontinence. J Urol 1989; 142: 512–515
9. Barett D M, Parulkar B G, Kramer S A. Experience with AS 800 artificial sphincter in pediatric and young adult patients. Urology 1993; 42: 431–436
10. Mitrofanoff P. Cystostomie continente trans-appendiculaire dans la traitement des vessies neurologiques. Chir Pediatr 1980; 21: 297–305
11. Duckett J W, Snyder H M. Continent urinary diversion: variation on the Mitrofanoff principle. J Urol 1986; 136: 58–62
12. Woodhouse C R J, Malone P R, Cumming J, Reilly T M. The Mitrofanoff principle for continent urinary diversion. Br J Urol 1989; 63: 53–57
13. Cedrou M, Gearhart J P. The Mitrofanoff principle: technique and application in continent urinary diversion. Urol Clin North Am 1991; 18: 615–621
14. Allen T D. The non-neurogenic neurogenic bladder. J Urol 1977; 117: 232
15. Mundy A R, Stephenson T P. 'Clam' ileocystoplasty for the treatment of refractory urge incontinence. Br J Urol 1985; 57: 641
16. Schwarz G R, Jeffs R D. Ileal conduit urinary diversion in children: computer analysis of follow-up from 2–16 years. J Urol 1975; 114: 285
17. Fisch M, Wammack R, Müller S C, Hohenfellner R. The Mainz pouch II. Eur Urol 1994; 25: 7–15
18. Horowitz M, Mitchell M E. The DAWG procedure, gastroplasty made better. J Urol 1994; 151: 1002
19. Elder J S. Continent appendicocolostomy: a variation of the Mitrofanoff principle in pediatric urinary tract reconstruction. J Urol 1992; 144: 117–119

The Monfort abdominoplasty for patients with prune belly syndrome

24

J. R. Woodard   T. S. Parrott
B. H. Broecker   E. A. Smith

Introduction

Prune belly syndrome is represented by the triad of urinary tract dilation, bilateral cryptorchidism and deficiency of the abdominal wall musculature. Although the grossly dilated urinary tract represents the greatest threat to the overall health of the individual, the physical appearance is dominated by a thin, lax and often severely wrinkled abdominal wall. The pathogenesis of this defect continues to stir debate. The pattern of the abdominal wall defect based on both electromyographic studies and anatomical observations is, however, well described and forms the basis of surgical correction. Generally, stronger electromyographic signals are found in the lateral and upper parts of the abdomen, with weak or absent responses in the suprapubic abdominal musculature.[1,2] Intraoperative findings mirror these studies, with hypoplasia of the medial portions of the lower transverse and oblique muscles and either more pronounced hypoplasia or aplasia of the suprapubic region of the rectus abdominis. Earlier operative descriptions were based on these observations and included resection of the most deficient muscle.[2] More recently, Ehrlich and Monfort have separately described operations in which the hypoplastic segments are spared and overlapped in a vertical fashion.[3,4] The authors' recent experience has involved use of the Monfort abdominoplasty.

Correction of the abdominal defect should be recognized as an important part of management. The patient achieves not only an obvious improvement in cosmetic appearance and psychological well-being but also may realize an improvement in bladder and bowel function. These potential benefits have been evaluated through patient interviews and urodynamic studies in the authors' first 12 patients undergoing the Monfort abdominoplasty.

Patients and methods

Surgical technique

The redundant abdominal wall tissue is tented up and the lines of incision from just inferior to the xiphoid to just superior to the symphysis pubis are delineated (Fig. 24.1a). Any asymmetry in the redundancy of the abdominal wall should be taken into account and the most lateral excursion of the incision is placed at the approximate level of the umbilicus to generate a more normal waist. A second circumscribing incision is planned to allow preservation of the umbilicus. The incisions are then formed and the intervening skin and dermis is excised (Fig. 24.1b). The abdominal cavity is entered sufficiently lateral to the rectus muscle to eliminate redundancy when the lateral edge of this incision is brought to the midline. The superior epigastric vessels superiorly and the inferior epigastric vessels inferiorly represent the surgical limits and they should be observed and protected before extending the incision (Fig. 24.1c). A central musculofascial plate with a reliable vascular supply is formed and sufficient transperitoneal access is provided to enable concomitant complex genitourinary procedures to be performed. Proceeding with the abdominoplasty, the parietal peritoneum overlying the lateral abdominal wall musculature is scored using the electrocautery (Fig. 24.2a). The edges of the central plate are sutured to the lateral abdominal musculature along this scored line and the two lateral flaps are brought over the central plate and sutured together in the midline (Fig. 24.2b). Closed suction drains are placed between the lateral flaps and the central plate. The umbilicus is brought up through this closure and finally the skin is reapproximated (Fig. 24.2c). A nasogastric tube and urethral Foley catheter are used during the initial postoperative period.

Since July 1991, 16 of the authors' patients have undergone abdominal wall remodelling after the technique of Monfort. The mean patient age at operation was 11 years (range 1.5–24 years). Urodynamic evaluation was performed preoperatively in the initial ten patients and in eight of these patients urodynamic studies were also completed after abdominoplasty. A detailed questionnaire regarding changes in bowel and bladder function was completed during follow-up visits by the initial twelve patients. Specifically, patients and their parents were asked to describe any positive or negative postoperative changes in the patient's bladder sensation, force of stream, voiding pattern and bowel habits. A voiding diary was kept over a course of 3 days and the preoperative and postoperative rates of culture-proven urinary tract infection (UTI) were compared.

(a)

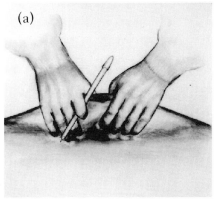

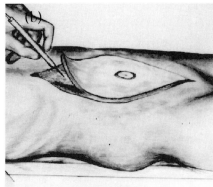

(c)

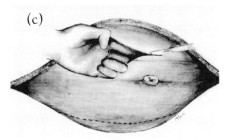

Figure 24.1. (a) Delineation of redundancy by tenting up abdominal wall. (b) Excision of skin (epidermis and dermis only) using electrocautery. Umbilicus is isolated with separate circumferential incision. (c) Abdominal wall central plate in incised at the lateral border of the 'rectus muscle' on either side, from the superior epigastric to inferior epigastric vessels, creating a central musculofascial plate.

Results

The authors' experience with the Monfort abdominoplasty now includes 16 patients, six of whom underwent additional complex procedures. When abdominoplasty alone was performed, the mean hospital stay was 7 days. Early postoperative complications have been limited to one case of transient breathing difficulty in the immediate postoperative period and one case of superficial wound dehiscence. The abdominal contour has been greatly improved in all patients and there has been uniform satisfaction with the postoperative result in both paediatric and adult patients. Although the follow-up period is less than 3 years for all patients, the contour of the repaired abdominal wall has been maintained.

Review of preoperative and postoperative urodynamics, voiding diaries and patient questionnaires reveals a trend toward improved voiding dynamics (Table 24.1). All patients demonstrated improved bladder sensation and post-voiding residual urine was reduced by 10–50%. Those patients that had required double voiding to promote bladder emptying found that this was necessary less often. Maximum detrusor pressures also tended to be higher. Overall, the incidence of UTI

(a)

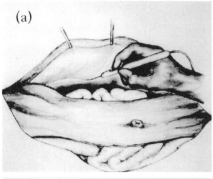

(b)

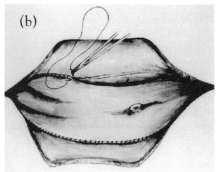

(c)

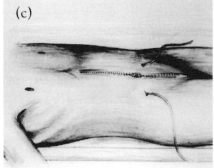

Figure 24.2. (a) Parietal peritoneum overlying the lateral abdominal wall musclature is scored using electrocautery. (b) Edges of the central plate are sutured to the lateral abdominal wall musculature along the scored line. (c) Lateral flaps are brought together in the midline with closed suction drains placed between the lateral flaps and the central plate. Skin is then brought together in the midline enveloping the previously isolated umbilicus.

Parameter	Preoperative	Postoperative
Maximum flow (ml/s)	16.3	17.4
Capacity*	2.1×	1.6×
Post-voiding residual (%)	40.3	13.0
Maximum detrusor pressure (cmH$_2$O)	62.1	62.3
Compliance (ml/cmH$_2$O)	192	93

*Expressed as a factor of the expected capacity for age.

Table 24.1. Results of urodynamic studies in 10 patients undergoing Monfort abdminoplasty

was reduced. The initial 12 patients as a group experienced 5.7 bouts of UTI per year and postoperatively this rate declined to 1.2 bouts per year. An improvement in bowel control with less constipation was reported in four patients.

Conclusions

Management of the abdominal wall defect in prune belly syndrome has been greatly aided by the development of vertical fascial overlapping abdominoplasty procedures. Previous reconstructive attempts, such as the Randolph abdominoplasty, achieved a reduction of the abdominal wall redundancy by full-thickness excision of the excess skin and fascia. Although the most deficient region of the abdominal wall had been identified and removed, the procedure provided no improvement in abdominal wall thickness or strength, and lateral bulging tended to remain uncorrected. The Monfort abdominoplasty accomplishes these goals and also provides a more normal contour at the waist.[5] Excellent results have also been reported with Ehrlich's procedure, which similarly exercises the principles of umbilical preservation and overlapping musculofascial flaps.[6] The reliable vascular pedicles serving the central fascial plate and the ability to leave the umbilicus undisturbed may represent relative advantages to the Monfort procedure. In addition, the Monfort procedure seems to facilitate transfer of the more substantial lateral musculature to the midline.

Although the majority of abdominoplasties performed by the authors have been in patients that were just prepubertal, an earlier age may be more suitable. As described by Monfort et al.,[4] the incisions allow for adequate access for concomitant genitourinary surgery and the procedure may be performed in infants. Certainly, earlier application provides for a more normal physique during the formative years. In addition to the cosmetic benefits, urodynamic evaluations have shown a trend towards improved bladder function. With improved bladder sensation and higher maximum detrusor pressures, voiding may become more complete. Subjective improvements in bowel control have also been reported. Complete investigation of all 16 patients is anticipated to verify further these encouraging early results.

References

1. Fallat M E, Skoog S J, Belman A B et al. The prune belly syndrome: a comprehensive approach to management. J Urol 1989; 142: 802–805
2. Randolph J G, Cavett C , Eng G. Surgical correction and rehabilitation for children with 'prune-belly ' syndrome. Ann Surg 1981; 193: 757–762
3. Erlich R M, Lesavoy M A, Fine R N. Total abdominal wall reconstruction in the prune-belly syndrome. J Urol 1986; 136: 282
4. Montfort G, Guys J M, Bocciardi A et al. A novel technique for reconstruction of the abdominal wall in the prune belly syndrome. J Urol 1991; 146: 639
5. Parrott T S, Woodard J R. The Montfort operation for abdominal wall reconstruction in the prune belly syndrome. J Urol 1992; 148: 688–690
6. Erlich R M, Levasoy M A. Umbilicus preservation with total abdominal wall reconstruction in prune belly syndrome. Urology 1993; 41: 231–232

25

Vaginoplasty with the bilateral labioscrotal flap: a new flap vaginoplasty

K. Nonomura   H. Kakizaki
T. Yamashita   Y. Asano   T. Koyanagi

Introduction

Flap vaginoplasty, the inverted U-shaped type originated by Fortunoff and coworkers in 1964,[1] has been applied worldwide to patients with masculinized female genitalia. Extensive experience with this procedure and technical advancements have afforded new surgical insight into its application. It should be limited to those cases in which the vaginal introitus is distal to the external urethral sphincter (low vaginal entry) and the most frequent complication is contraction of the new vaginal introitus, which occurs as a result of ischaemic and fibrotic changes in the overlapping suture line between the flap and posterior vaginal wall. Maintenance of a good blood supply for the flap and tension-free anastomosis should always be kept in mind to avoid this complication. From the technical surgical viewpoint, the authors used a bilateral labioscrotal flap (M-shaped flap) instead of the inverted U-shaped flap because the labioscrotal skin is more elastic and more easily elongated than the perineal skin. This chapter reports the results of their experience using this M-shaped flap.

Patients and methods

Patients

From January 1985 to December 1993, 20 children underwent feminizing genitoplasty in the authors' clinic. M-shaped flap vaginoplasty was used for 14 patients with the low vaginal entry (Table 25.1). At the time of vaginoplasty they ranged from 2 to 17 years (median 4.5 years) of age. Nine with congenital adrenal hyperplasia (CAH), whose ages ranged from 2 to 5 years with a mean of 3.2 years, underwent total genital reconstruction (clitolabiovaginoplasty) as a primary definitive one-stage repair. Another two with CAH, aged 16 and 17 years, underwent

Diagnosis	No. of patients	Age at operation (years)	Surgical procedure
CAH*	11		
	9	2-5 (mean 3.2)	Clitolabiovaginoplasty
	2	16, 17	Revision of vaginal stenosis
MGD†	2	2, 10	Gonadectomy and clitolabiovaginoplasty
MPH‡	1	13	Excision of vaginal septum and clitolabiovaginoplasty
Total	14	Median 4.5	

*CAH, Congenital adrenal hyperplasia; †MGD, mixed gonadal dysgenesis; ‡MPH, male pseudohermaphroditism.

Table 25.1. Details of patients undergoing vaginoplasty with the bilateral labioscrotal flap

vaginoplasty alone for stenosis of the vaginal introitus after the previous genitoplasties. In two children aged 2 and 10 years, with mixed gonadal dysgenesis, total genital reconstruction was performed simultaneously following gonadectomy. In a 13-year-old girl with dysgenetic male pseudohermaphroditism, the vaginoplasty followed endoscopic excision of the vaginal septum.

The genetics, hormonal response and anatomical status of all patients with ambiguous genitalia were evaluated and the diagnosis was made before genital reconstruction. Eleven children with CAH had the normal 46XX karyotype genetically and 21-hydroxylase deficiency endocrinologically. Another three children with gonadal dysgenesis had a Y chromosome, so that the gonads were ultimately removed when it was decided to raise them as females.

Surgical technique

The child is placed in the dorsal lithotomy position. Intraoperative endoscopy is routinely performed using an 8–10 Fr infantile panendoscope to determine the distance to the urogenital sinus, whether the entrance of the vagina is located distal to the external urethral sphincter, and the existence of the portio vaginalis. When the entrance of the vagina is found, two different small catheters are passed to the vaginal cavity and to the bladder under direct vision; this endoscopic preparation facilitates the following surgical procedure (Fig. 25.1).

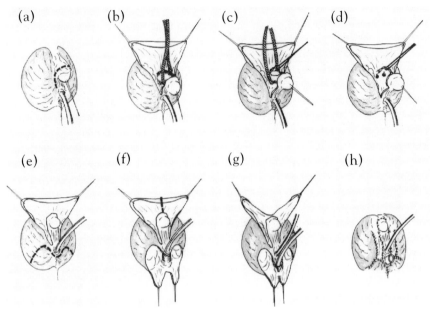

Figure 25.1. Clitolabiovaginoplasty. (a) The broken line outlines the semicircumcoronal incision of the clitoral recession. A Foley catheter is placed in the vaginal cavity. (b) Degloving the clitoral body circumferentially. (c) Isolation of the neurovascular bundles of the clitoris. (d) Resection of the corpus cavernosum without the neurovascular bundles and glans clitoris. (e) After the glans clitoris has been anchored to the mons pubis, a bilateral labioscrotal flap is designed for vaginoplasty (the broken line). (f) Elevation of labioscrotal flaps and dissection of the surrounding tissues from the urogenital sinus posteriorly. The dorsal foreskin is bivalved for labioplasty. (g) Incision of the rear wall of the urogenital sinus and vaginal introitus in the midline. A urethral catheter is placed in the bladder if this has not been done at step (a). Bilateral labioscrotal flaps are approximated and sutured together. Bisected dorsal foreskin flaps are ready to be advanced downwards to create the labium minor. (h) The labioscrotal flap is inlayed and sutured to the posterolateral vaginal wall. Dorsal foreskin flaps are draped around the glans clitoris towards the new vaginal introitus and meet the ipsilateral labioscrotal flap. A urethral catheter and a vaginal prosthesis are in place.

The clitoral recession technique is employed in the standard manner used for clitoplasty. A traction suture is placed on the glans clitoris. The incision for clitoplasty is along the dorsal sulcus coronalis of the glans clitoris and runs laterally on the medial border of the bilateral labioscrotal folds, extending to the level of the opening of the urogenital sinus (Fig. 25.1a). A sharp skin incision is made with fine curved iris scissors. The dorsal foreskin is detached from the clitoral body for the further labioplasty (Fig. 25.1b). After the clitoral body has been degloved, the dorsal neurovascular bundles are isolated from the corpus cavernosum (Fig. 25.1c). The corpus cavernosum is amputated and removed between a point just proximal to the glans and a point just distal to the crus clitoridis while preserving the neurovascular bundles (Fig 25.1d). The glans clitoris is anchored underneath the symphysis pubis.

The bilateral labioscrotal flap is then designed for vaginoplasty. This M-shaped skin incision extends along the opening of the urogenital sinus in the midline and laterally to the lower one-third of the labioscrotal folds (Figs 25.1e, 25.2a, 25.3a). The bilateral flaps are elevated with thick and vascular-rich subcutaneous tissues. The ventral portion of the urogenital sinus is freed from surrounding subcutaneous tissue (Fig. 25.1f). The vertical incision at the 6 o'clock position of the urogenital sinus is made to reach the vaginal introitus. Both medial edges of the labioscrotal flaps are approximated by interrupted two-layer sutures (Figs 25.1g, 25.2b). The distance of the approximation is adjusted in accordance with the depth of the incised vaginal introitus (Figs 25.1h, 25.2c). This flap is inlayed as one body and anastomosed in two layers to the posterior edge of the vaginal introitus with as little tension as possible. For these meticulous sutures, 5/0 or 6/0 absorbable stitches are usually used. The lateral sites of the flap are sutured to adjacent skin edges of labioscrotal folds.

After completion of this vaginal exteriorization the dorsal clitoral foreskin is bisected in the midline in the manner of the Byars flap (Fig. 25.1g). The divided skin flaps are wrapped around the recessed clitoris and advanced caudolaterally on the ipsilateral side to create labia minora. The most caudal portion of the flaps is set to suture to the most cranial portion of each labioscrotal flap (Fig. 25.1h). Penrose drains are placed in bilateral labioscrotal subcutaneous spaces before the skin closure is completed.

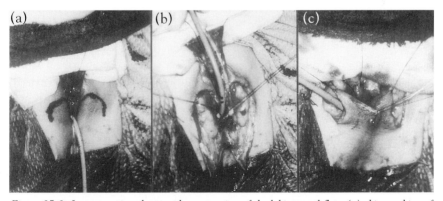

Figure 25.2. Intraoperative photographs at creation of the labioscrotal flap: (a) skin marking of the labioscrotal flap using gentian violet after anchoring the glans clitoris; (b) elevation of the bilateral labioscrotal flaps; traction sutures are placed on each flap and the edges of the incised urogenital sinus; (c) approximation of bilateral labioscrotal flaps in two layers.

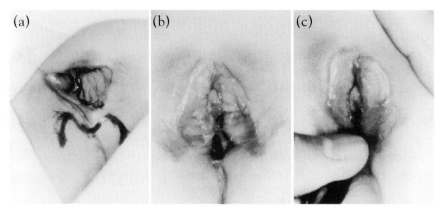

Figure 25.3. Pre- and postoperative photographs in a 2-year-old patient with congenital adrenal hyperplasia: (a) traction suture on the glans clitoris and skin marking for clitolabiovaginoplasty; (b, c) month 3 after operation; a metal bougie (30 Fr) is easily introduced.

A Foley catheter is left indwelling in the bladder for 5–7 days. An appropriately sized vaginal prosthesis is also left in the vaginal cavity and a compressive surgical dressing is applied for 2 or 3 days.

Results

In the first case, careless rough bites at skin closure caused a minor dog-ear deformity of the major labium. For the other 13 children satisfactory cosmetic results were achieved (Fig. 25.3b). The vaginal introitus was initially calibrated 2–3 months after surgery. This regular periodic calibration was carried out every 6–12 months until self-calibration was possible (Fig. 25.3c). Vaginal stenosis did not occur in any patient.

Discussion

In the past three decades there have been various technical improvements in feminizing genitoplasty. In terms of clitoral enlargement total amputation has been abandoned and relocation and plication of the clitoral body has been developed.[2] In addition, subtotal or segmental resection preserving the glans clitoris and its neurovascular bundles has been popularized as a standard clitoplasty procedure. The dorsal clitoral foreskin is now used not only to wrap the recessed glans but also to create the minor labium.[3] This procedure gives satisfactory cosmetic and functional results.

Meanwhile, vaginal reconstruction depends on the anatomical variations of individual ambiguous genitalia. If a vagina is absent or too small, vaginal substitution such as enterovaginoplasty should be considered. If a capacious vagina exists, the location of its introitus determines the surgical procedure. Fortunately, it is located distal to the external urethral sphincter in the majority of cases of female pseudohermaphroditism and mixed gonadal dysgenesis, so that flap vaginoplasty can be undertaken at the time of clitolabioplasty. Although high vaginal entry just beneath or proximal to the external urethral sphincter is rare, flap vaginoplasty should be avoided in this case. Flap vaginoplasty in the presence of high vaginal entry risks transection of the external urethral sphincter, with subsequent stress incontinence. Moreover, severe female hypospadias also makes the patient wet and prone to infection from voided urine entrapped in the vagina. In such cases pull-through vaginoplasty with the urethra preserved should be selected.[3,4] This is why endoscopic evaluation of these anatomical relationships is important.

Those surgeons who employ flap vaginoplasty with a perineal U-shaped flap emphasize the elevation of a wide-based and well-vascularized flap.[5,6] However, posteromedian perineal skin is usually fibrotic and lacks elasticity. The authors have used an M-shaped flap, as originated by Hecker in 1985,[7] to avoid these weak points of the perineal flap,[8] although the base of the flap is still derived from narrow perineal skin. The base of the flap has been modified to extend the bilateral labioscrotal folds. Additionally, approximation of the bilateral labioscrotal flaps in accordance with the distance to the 6 o'clock position of the vaginal introitus enables the elastic subcutaneous tissue of the labioscrotal folds to be inlaid to the suture line without undue tension. A similar surgical technique was recently reported in a case of mixed gonadal dysgenesis.[9] These facts make the labioscrotal flap more suitable than the traditional perineal flap as the optimal flap for vaginoplasty, although the long-term outcome is not yet clear.

No patient so far has developed vaginal contracture, as determined by periodic calibration of the vagina. Until finger calibration by the patient or sexual intercourse can be accomplished, calibration on follow-up is indispensable even for the most successful flap vaginoplasty. In the authors' experience, regular calibration every 6–12 months, with the first at month 3 after operation, appear to be optimal.

References

1. Fortunoff S, Latimer J K, Edson M. Vaginoplasty technique for female pseudohermaphrodites. Surg Gynecol Obstet 1964; 118: 545–548
2. Lattimer J K. Relocation and recession of the enlarged clitoris with preservation of the glans: An alternative to amputation. J Urol 1961; 86: 113–116
3. Hendren W H, Donahoe P K. Correction of congenital abnormalities of the vagina and perineum. J Pediatr Surg 1980; 15: 751–763

4. Gonzalez R, Fernandes E T. Single-stage feminization genitoplasty. J Urol 1990; 143: 776–778

5. Perlmutter A D. Adrenogenital syndrome. In: Glenn J F (ed) Urologic surgery, 3rd ed. Philadelphia: Lippincott, 1986: 1043–1052

6. Donahoe P K, Hendren W H. Perineal reconstruction in ambiguous genitalia infants raised as females. Ann Surg 1984; 200: 363–371

7. Hecker W C. Correction of clitoral hypertrophy and urogenital sinus with low vaginal entry. Surgical correction of intersexual genitalia and female genital malformation. Berlin: Springer-Verlag, 1985: 28–46

8. Asano Y, Nonomura K, Koyanagi T. The experience of feminizing genitoplasty. Jpn J Pediatr Surg 1991; 27: 1153–1158 (in Japanese)

9. Sheldon C A, Gilbert A, Lewis A. Vaginal reconstruction: clinical technical principles. J Urol 1994; 152: 190–195

Syndrome of early urethral obstruction: a lethal entity?

26

J. de Vries   M. de Wildt   W. Feitz
J. Nijhuis

Introduction

In the last two decades, prenatal ultrasound screening has increased to the extent that it is performed at least once during most pregnancies. Consequently, the diagnosis of foetal abnormalities has increased: for example, hydronephrosis is the most common finding in 50% of foetal abnormalities detected by ultrasound investigation.[1] Since the beginning of the 1980s many studies have been dedicated to the different findings of foetal urological abnormalities and their postnatal outcome (e.g. renal agenesis, multicystic kidneys, hydronephrosis, ureteropelvic junction obstruction, megaureter, megacystis, prune belly syndrome, vesicoureteral reflux and other deformities of the urinary tract).[2-4] In 50–78% of cases the prenatal diagnosis is confirmed postnatally.[5-7]

The first case report of a prenatally diagnosed congenital obstructive uropathy, describing an enormously dilated bladder at an early stage of pregnancy, was published in 1983 by Korenromp et al;[8] they also described the fatal outcome and the autopsy findings. From week 12 of gestation the foetal bladder can be visualized by ultrasound in 50% of cases.[9] The size of the bladder changes because the foetus empties its bladder every 30–40 min.[10] A prolonged or repeated ultrasound investigation should be performed where visualization of the bladder is difficult. When a lower urinary tract obstruction is present, the bladder wall, which is normally thin, becomes clearly visible owing to hypertrophy. If, because of vesicoureteral reflux or an obstruction at the ureteral or bladder level, the ureters and kidneys are involved, a massive dilatation can often be seen. Depending on the gestational age at which the obstruction occurs and on the severity of the obstruction, the negative effect of kidney development can be very pronounced.

In the past 4 years the authors have encountered eight cases, presenting themselves as extreme dilatation of the foetal bladder in early pregnancy without pronounced or noticeable dilatation of the upper urinary tract. Because of its poor prognosis, this early urethral obstruction syndrome (EUOS) appears to represent a lethal entity in the spectrum of foetal obstructive uropathies.

Patients and methods

Between September 1989 and November 1993 the authors encountered eight pregnancies with signs of a low-level obstructive uropathy. These pregnancies were referred to the prenatal diagnostic centre, either because of a suspicion of congenital abnormalities on sonography or because of an increased risk of foetal abnormality in view of the patients' (family) history. Sonographic investigation in these eight cases showed a large transsonity in the foetal abdomen. The mean gestational age at first presentation of this abnormality was 15 weeks (range 12–24 weeks). The examinations were all performed by an obstetrician experienced in prenatal ultrasound screening and these abnormalities were discussed by a multidisciplinary team consisting of an obstetrician, neonatologist, geneticist, paediatric urologist, paediatric surgeon, social worker, medical ethics specialist and a representative of the nursing staff.

In four of these cases of EUOS, percutenous puncture of the foetal bladder was performed: in one case a vesicoamniotic shunt was placed and in the remaining three cases a conservative approach was chosen.

A transabdominal placental biopsy was performed in six cases, and in one case a cordocentesis was performed for rapid karyotyping.

Results

The outcome of the prenatal findings, the management and postmortem diagnosis in the eight cases is outlined below and summarized in Table 26.1 and Table 26.2.

Case 1

The first ultrasound examination at a gestational age (GA) of 8 weeks showed no abnormalities. An ultrasound examination at 12 weeks showed a transsonity in the abdomen with a diameter of 1.3 cm. Both kidneys had a dysplastic aspect and the lungs appeared to be hypoplastic, based on the thoracic and foetal abdominal circumference ratio (TC/FAC ratio). A curettage was performed at 13 weeks. Because of the fragmentation of the material, necropsy could not give any conclusive answers.

Case 2

An ultrasound examination at a GA of 12 weeks revealed no abnormalities. A second sonographic investigation at 19 weeks showed two large abdominal transsonities, 7 and 3 cm in diameter. The thoracic circumference was very small and there was an oligohydramnios present. No other organs in the abdomen were recognizable. The foetal bladder was punctured for urinary analysis. At 20 weeks, the pregnancy was terminated. Autopsy showed a massively dilated bladder that extended into the right thorax. Atresia of the urethra was seen, with agenesis of the left kidney and ureter. The right kidney appeared to be normal. Concomitant non-urological malformations comprised anal atresia and a neural tube defect.

Case 3

An ultrasound examination was performed at a GA of 14 weeks, which revealed a cystic process in the abdomen (2 cm in diameter). Karyotyping after chorionic villi sampling revealed trisomy 18 (47,XY + 18). One week later the foetal bladder was punctured for urinary analysis. At 16 weeks the pregnancy was terminated. On autopsy no connection was found between the atretic urethra and the bladder. The kidney pelvices showed no signs of dilatation. All other internal organs were apparently normal.

Case 4

Routine ultrasonography at a GA of 14 weeks was normal. The second sonographic investigation at 24 weeks now showed an enlarged bladder with a diameter of 3–4 cm with a hypertrophic bladder wall 0.5 cm thick (Fig. 26.1). The severe oligohydramnios made it difficult to visualize the kidneys, but there were no clear signs of dilatation.

This case was extensively discussed by the authors' multidisciplinary team and after ample consultation with the parents it was decided to place a vesicoamniotic shunt. Before this procedure an artificial amniotic fluid compartment was created with a salt solution and thereafter both kidneys appeared to have a dysplastic aspect. A pigtail catheter was put into the bladder and left as a shunt to the amniotic cavity. During the first 2 weeks the thoracic diameter increased and the amount of amniotic fluid became normal. However, at 27 weeks a premature delivery occurred and the child died 1 h after birth. Autopsy revealed a narrow but passable urethra. The bladder was extremely dilated, with hypertrophy and trabeculation. The pigtail proved to be lying in the bladder without connection to the amniotic cavity. The upper urinary tract showed an image of polycystic kidneys with dilatation of both the pyelocalyceal system and the ureters.

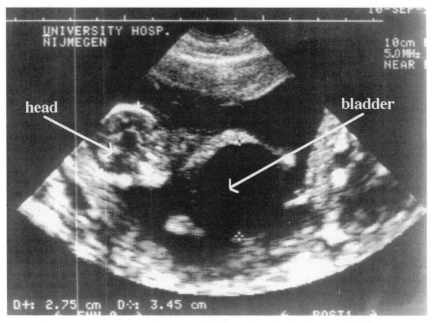

Figure 26.1. Case 4: ultrasound image (week 24) of the foetal abdomen and head, showing the enormous bladder compared with the size of the head.

Case 5

A first ultrasound examination at a GA of 15 weeks showed severe abnormalities as the complete abdomen was filled with an enlarged bladder. At 16 weeks, the pregnancy was terminated. Autopsy showed an enormously dilated bladder with a thin abdominal wall. There were no signs of hydroureteronephrosis. Microscopic examination of the kidneys showed small cysts (Potter type IV). The lungs were hypoplastic.

Case 6

The first ultrasound examination at a GA of 12 weeks revealed an abdominal cystic lesion with a diameter of 3 cm. The foetal bladder was punctured for urinalysis. Because of the suspected bad prognosis, the pregnancy was terminated. Unfortunately, the foetus was damaged by the procedure to such an extent that no conclusive diagnosis could be made. Only microscopic examination of renal tissue showed cystic lesions (Potter type IV).

Case 7

On the first ultrasonography at a GA of 16 weeks, a huge transsonity was seen in the foetal abdomen. The kidneys could not be visualized. After

140 ml urine had been removed, the bladder showed a very trabeculated image. On sonographic follow-up the bladder filled again, so two more bladder punctures were performed, 7 and 13 days after the first. The kidneys were clearly visible and showed some hydronephrosis. Thirty minutes after a premature birth at 27 weeks' gestation the girl died because of respiratory difficulties. On autopsy there were signs of a persistent cloacal membrane with complete atresia of the urethra, anus and vagina. The abdomen had a prune belly aspect and there was hydroureteronephrosis on both sides. Non-urological deformities included malrotation of the intestines and hypoplasia of the lungs.

Case 8

At a GA of 12 weeks a routine sonographic investigation was performed, which showed a cystic lesion 12 mm in diameter in the foetal bladder region. Repeated ultrasound investigations revealed increasing size of the foetal bladder, with a thick bladder wall (0.3–0.6 cm) and mild hydroureteronephrosis on the right side. The amount of amniotic fluid was decreasing. At 15 weeks the pregnancy was terminated because of the lethal prognosis. Autopsy showed a dilated bladder with urethral atresia. The left kidney revealed hydronephrosis with dilated calyces and pseudocystic lesions at the renal surface. The right kidney had a similar aspect and was for a large part shrunken. The testicles were normal and located in the abdomen. There was hypoplasia of the lungs; furthermore, there was anal and rectal atresia and the distal colon was dilated.

Characteristic	Case no.							
	1	2	3	4	5	6	7	8
Gestation age at first presentation	12	19	14	24	15	12	15	12
Karyotype	–	46,XY	47,XY	46,XY	46,XY	46,XY	46,XY	46,XY
Oligohydramnios	No	Yes	Yes	Yes	Yes	No	Yes	Yes
Hydro(uretero)- nephrosis	No	No	No	Yes	No	No	Yes	Yes
Dysplastic aspect of kidneys on US	Yes	No	No	Yes	No	No	No	No
Hypertrophic bladder wall	No	No	No	Yes	No	No	Yes	Yes

Table 26.1. Characteristics of eight cases of early urethral obstruction syndrome

| | Case no. | | | | | | | |
Finding	1	2	3	4	5	6	7	8
Urethral atresia	?	+	+	+	+/-	?	+	+
Anal atresia	?	+	-	-	-	?	+	+
Hydro(uretero)nephrosis	?	-	-	+	-	?	+	+
Pulmonary hypoplasia	?	+	-	+	+	?	+	+
Malrotation of intestines	?	-	-	-	-	?	+	-
Thin abdominal wall	?	-	-	-	+	?	+	-
Neural tube defect	?	+	-	-	-	?	-	-
Cystic kidney	?	-	-	+	+	+	-	+

Table 26.2. Early urethral obstruction syndrome: findings on autopsy

Discussion

The syndrome of early urethral obstruction is characterized by the following features. There is a massive hypertrophic bladder distension at the end of the first trimester of pregnancy, with little, if any, dilatation of the upper urinary tract. There is an anatomical obstruction at the level of the urethra, caused either by urethral atresia, by severely obstructive posterior urethral valves or by a persistent cloacal membrane.[11] The kidneys can show signs of renal dysplasia. There is oligohydramnios, which causes pulmonary hypoplasia. There is a male predominance with no maldevelopment of internal or external genitalia. In the case of a female foetus, other congenital deformities can be present. In the authors' eight cases of EUOS, concomitant non-urological malformations were anal atresia, neural tube defect and trisomy 18.

If, on prenatal ultrasound examination, dilatation of the foetal urinary tract is found, questions about diagnosis and management can be raised. The main goal must be to preserve as much renal function as possible. Where loss of renal function is suspected, in the presence of severe dilatation, for example, the damage is probably already done. Prognosis for the future function should be the issue. In this context it still has to be proved whether any renal function can be saved by early removal of obstruction. In cases 2 and 3, no dysplasia was found despite the early obstruction. In cases 5 and 6, with only slight dilatation, cystic dysplasia was seen at autopsy.

In experimental settings the role of obstruction of the urinary tract in subsequent dilatation of the collecting system and renal dysplasia has been debated. It has been stated that the development of renal dysplasia depends on the time at which obstruction occurs: an early obstruction causes dysplastic kidneys; if obstruction occurs later in pregnancy it causes hydronephrosis.[12–14] However, it is still not clear whether the presence of dysplastic kidneys, which is seen in obstructive uropathy, is caused by the obstruction or is the result of a disorder in the development of the kidney itself.

Analysis of foetal urine after puncture of the foetal bladder to determine the tubular function might enable the assessment of the amount of renal damage to be assessed. The composition of normal foetal urine is probably constant and related to the duration of the pregnancy. With good renal function, hypotonic urine is formed; where renal function is impaired, the foetal kidney acts as a salt-loser and isotonic urine is formed. If the results of ultrasound, showing severe oligohydramnios and signs of cystic kidneys, are combined with the results of foetal bladder puncture with sodium values of over 100 mEq, choride values of more than 90 mEq and an osmolarity of more than 210 mosmol, the prognosis for the foetus is poor.[15] A high concentration of beta-2 microglobulin seems to correlate with poor renal function but the specificity and sensitivity are low and age-controlled normal values are not yet available.[16] All four cases in which urine was obtained had more than one parameter with a prognostic poor value.

One of the possible ways of preventing further damage to the kidneys and of preventing pulmonary hypoplasia is to shunt the urinary tract with the amniotic cavity. Although there is a survival rate of 50%, this procedure has not been shown to be beneficial because of the high neonatal death rate in the surviving group (97%), with pulmonary hypoplasia as the main cause.[17,18] One of the technical problems can be displacement of the shunting catheter, so that there is no further drainage of amniotic fluid, as seen in case 4. If obstruction is already present at an early stage of pregnancy (EUOS), shunting is not a desirable option.

An obstruction of the urinary tract as early as in EUOS causes oligohydramnios at an early stage; development of pulmonary hypoplasia is therefore inevitable. The authors postulate, therefore, that EUOS is a lethal form of obstructive uropathy that can be caused either by urethral atresia, by severely obstructive posterior urethral valves or by persistence of the cloacal membrane. Taking also in consideration the bad prognostic signs of loss of renal function and the poor results of invasive intrauterine intervention, termination of the pregnancy at an early stage appears to be justified.

References

1. Blyth B, Snyder H M, Duckett J W. Antenatal diagnosis and subsequent management of hydronephrosis. J Urol 1993; 149: 693–698
2. Reuss A, Wladimiroff J W, Scholtmeijer R J et al. Prenatal evaluation and outcome of fetal obstructive uropathies. Prenatal Diagn 1988; 8: 93–102
3. Furlong L A, Williamson R A, Bonsib S et al. Pregnancy outcome following ultrasound diagnosis of fetal urinary tract anomalies and/or oligohydramnios. Fetal Ther 1986; I: 134–145
4. Ransley P G, Dhillon H K, Gordon I et al. The postnatal management of hydronephrosis diagnosed by prenatal ultrasound. J Urol 1990; 144: 584–587
5. Sholder A J, Maizels M, Depp R et al. Caution in antenatal intervention. J Urol 1988; 139: 1026–1029
6. Scott J E, Renwick M. Antenatal diagnosis of congenital abnormalities in the urinary tract. Br J Urol 1988; 62: 295–300
7. Livera L N, Brookfield D S, Egginton J A, Hawnaur J M. Antenatal ultrasonography to detect fetal renal abnormalities: a prospective screening programe. Br Med J 1989; 298: 1421
8. Korenromp M J, Stassen M J, van Ertbruggen I, Kriek R. The natural course of early intrauterine urethral obstruction. Am J Obstet Gynecol 1983; 147: 465–466
9. Green J J, Hobbins J C. Abdominal ultrasound examination of the first-trimester fetus. Am J Obstet Gynecol 1988; 159: 165–175
10. Wladimiroff J W, Campbell S. Fetal urine-production rates in normal and complicated pregnancy. Lancet 1974; 1: 151–154
11. Lyons Jones K. Early urethral obstruction sequence. In: Smith D W (ed) Smith's recognisable patterns of human malformation. Philadelphia: Saunders, 1988: 562–563
12. McVary K T, Maizels M. Urinary obstruction reduces glomerulogenesis in the developing kidney: a model in the rabbit. J Urol 1989; 142: 646–651
13. Peters C A, Carr M C, Lais A et al. The response of the fetal kidney to obstruction. J Urol 1992; 148: 503–509
14. Ward R M, Starr N T, Snow B W et al. Serial renal function in an ovine model of unilateral fetal urinary tract obstruction. J Urol 1989; 142: 652–656
15. Glick R L, Harrison M R, Golbus M S et al. Management of the fetus with congenital hydronephrosis II: prognostic criteria and selection for treatment. J Pediatr Surg 1985; 20: 376–387
16. Burhard R, Gordjani N, Bald R. Protein analysis in amniotic fluid and fetal urine for the assessment of fetal renal function and dysfunction. Fetal Ther 1987; 2: 188–196
17. Manning F A, Harrison M R, Rodeck C. Catheter shunts for fetal hydronephrosis and hydrocephalus. New Engl J Med 1986; 315: 336–340
18. Elder J S, Ducket J W Jr, Snyder H M. Intervention for fetal obstructive uropathy: has it been effective? Lancet 1987; 1007–1010

Index